AF872739

The Garden Cure

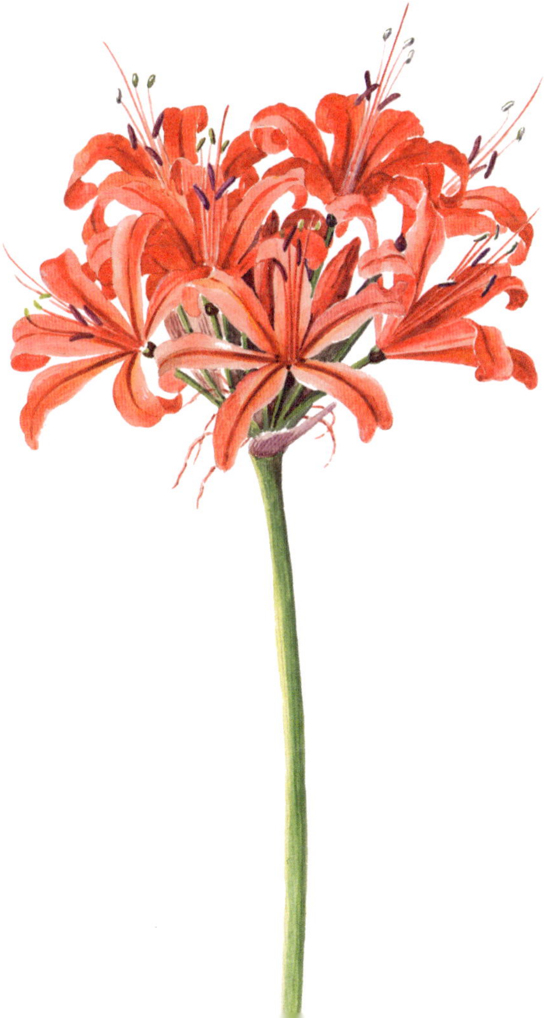

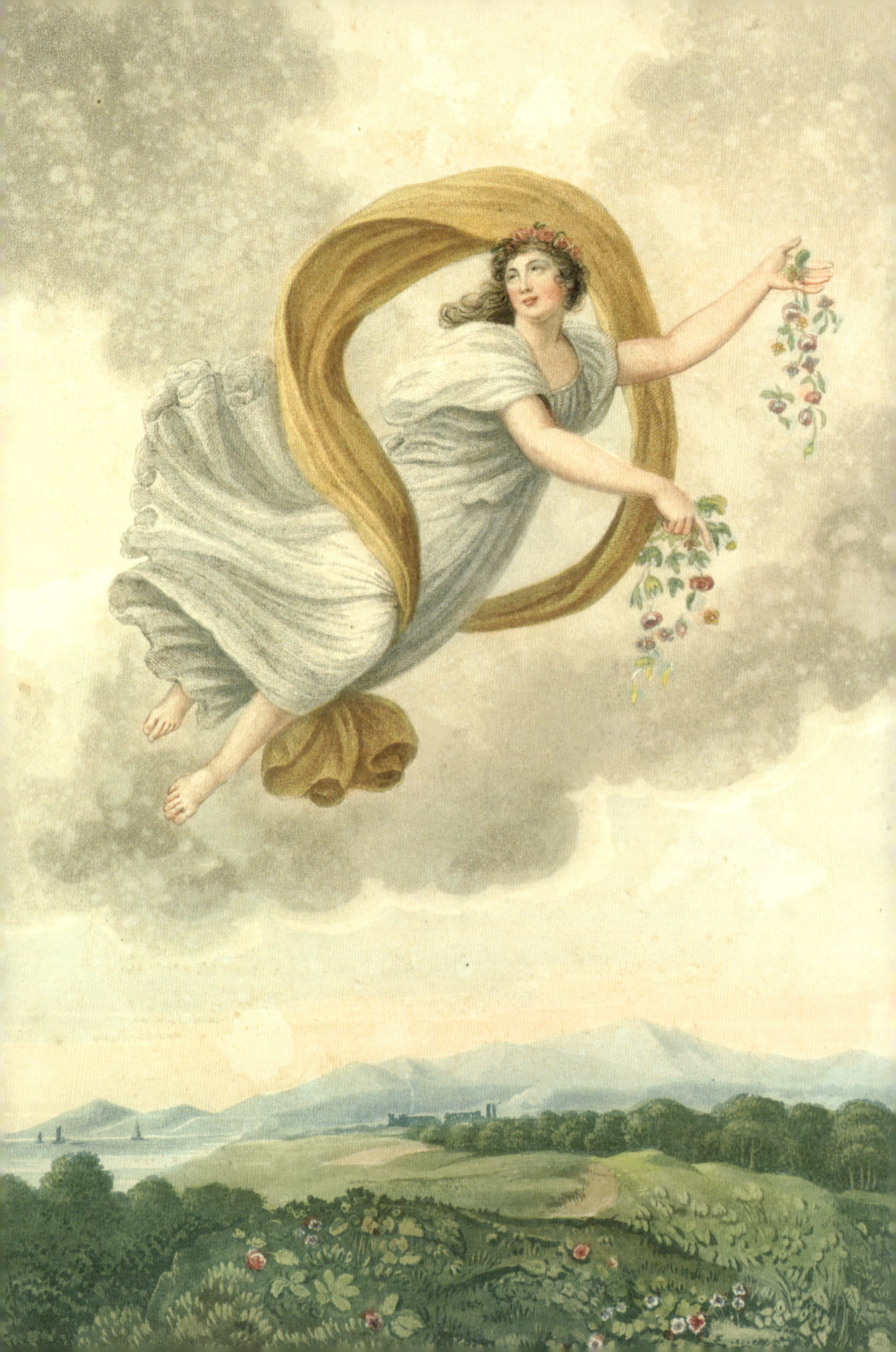

RHS

The Garden Cure

100 Remarkable Remedies for the Curious Gardener

Ann Treneman

MITCHELL BEAZLEY

Contents

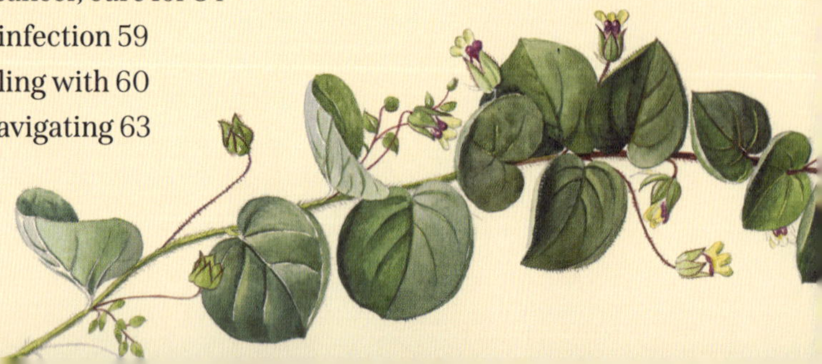

Chapter 3

SPIRIT

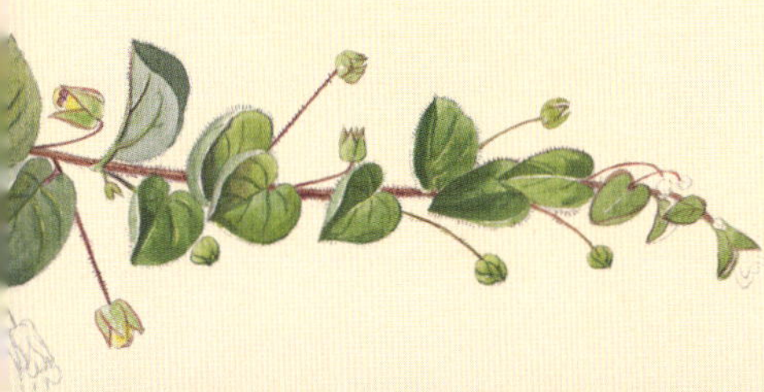

Chapter 4

LIFE

Introduction

Imagine you could go into an apothecary and, instead of seeing rows of jars with their cures, there was a display of all the plants from which they came. You'd be able to point down to a tiny snowdrop or up to a very large horse chestnut tree (it's a giant cabinet). There would be an entire herbaceous border, sweet peas and roses, daisies and foxgloves. On the shady bottom shelf, there would be an array of frogs and snails and even, possibly, puppy dog tails as dogs love a garden cure too.

That is what I imagined while putting together this most unusual apothecary's cabinet of a book. It's a thoroughly modern (and sumptuously illustrated) herbal that deals with problems of all kinds for the body, mind and the always important spirit. Many ailments or dilemmas are serious, others whimsical and then there are those that spring from the kind of lives we lead now. Sex, death, life and an overwhelming desire to hear beautiful music: there's a garden cure in this book for all of us.

It's been fascinating to explore how plant cures were discovered and I have been struck by how, time and again, it was a combination of serendipity and the appliance of science that saved the day. The scientists and researchers may not be household names but some of their cures are. This is why there is space, in our magical apothecary cabinet, to celebrate those unsung plant detectives who refused to give up on their quest to cure. They have saved, and enhanced, millions of lives. Now when I see a snowdrop, I know that it's much more than just a beautiful flower.

Ann Treneman

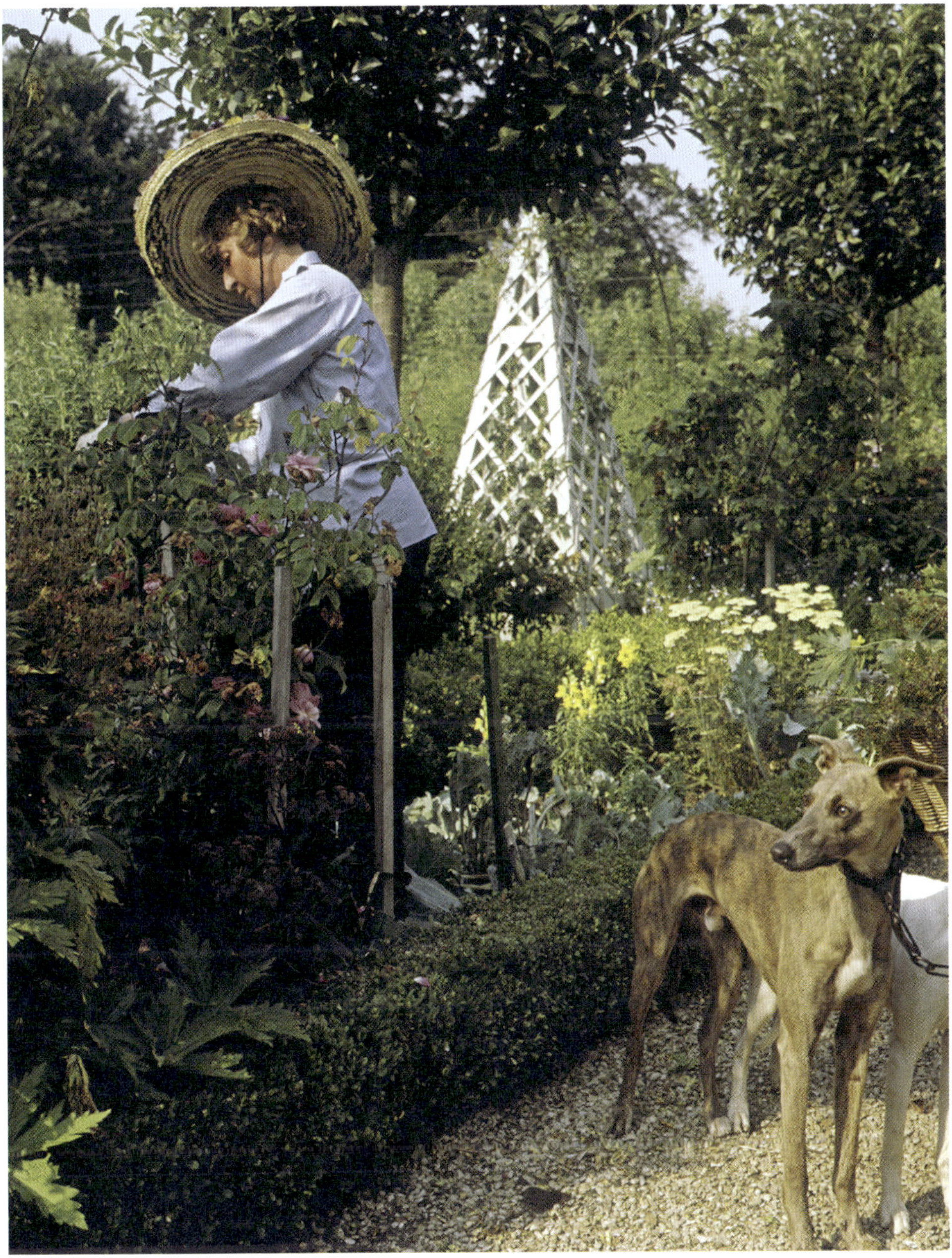

A garden meditation: designer Nancy Lancaster and her dogs at her Haseley Court home, Oxfordshire, photographed by Valerie Finnis in the 1950s.

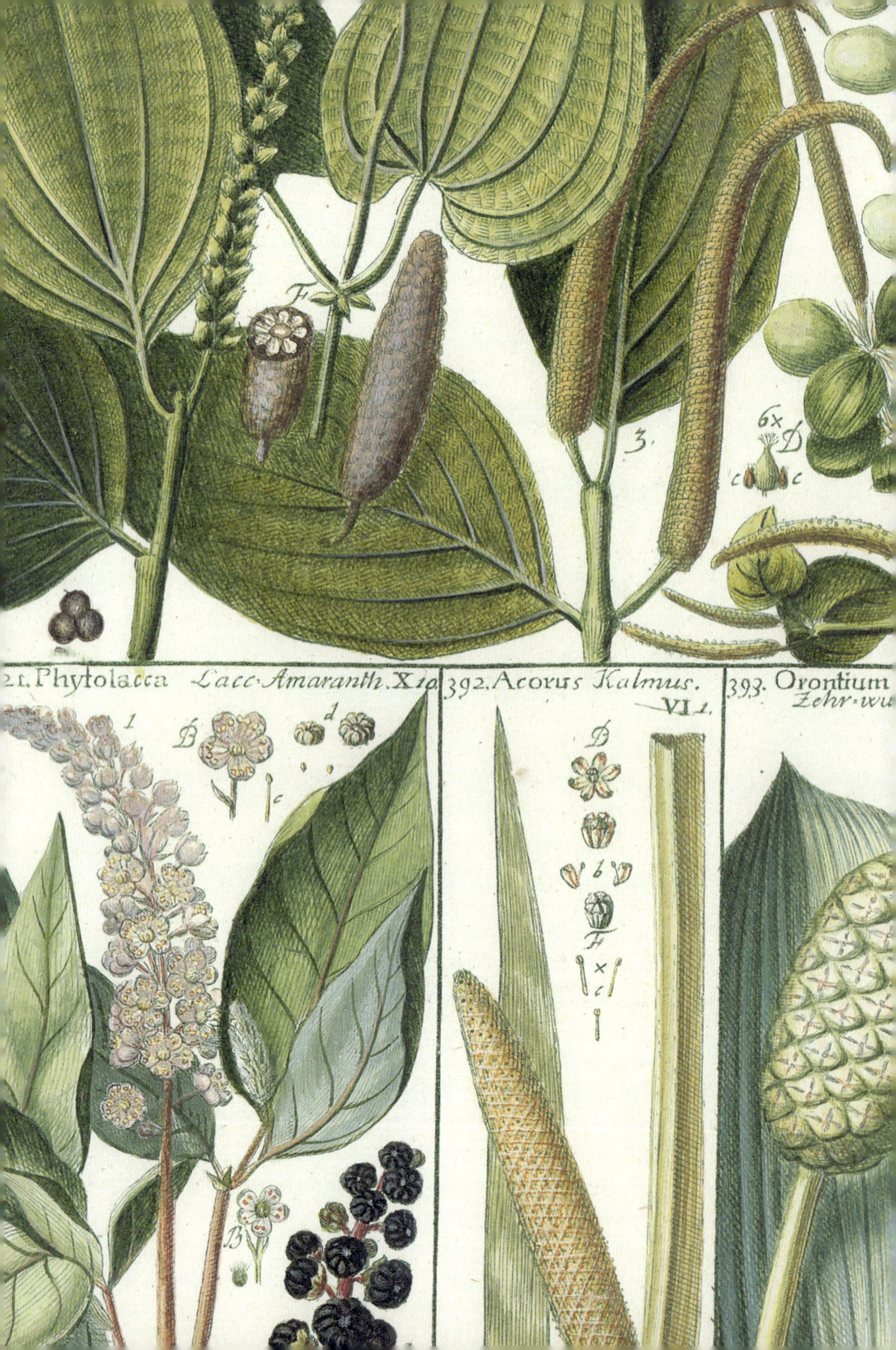

3.
21. Phytolacca Lacc-Amaranth. X 10.
392. Acorus Kalmus. VI 1.
393. Orontium
Zehr-wu

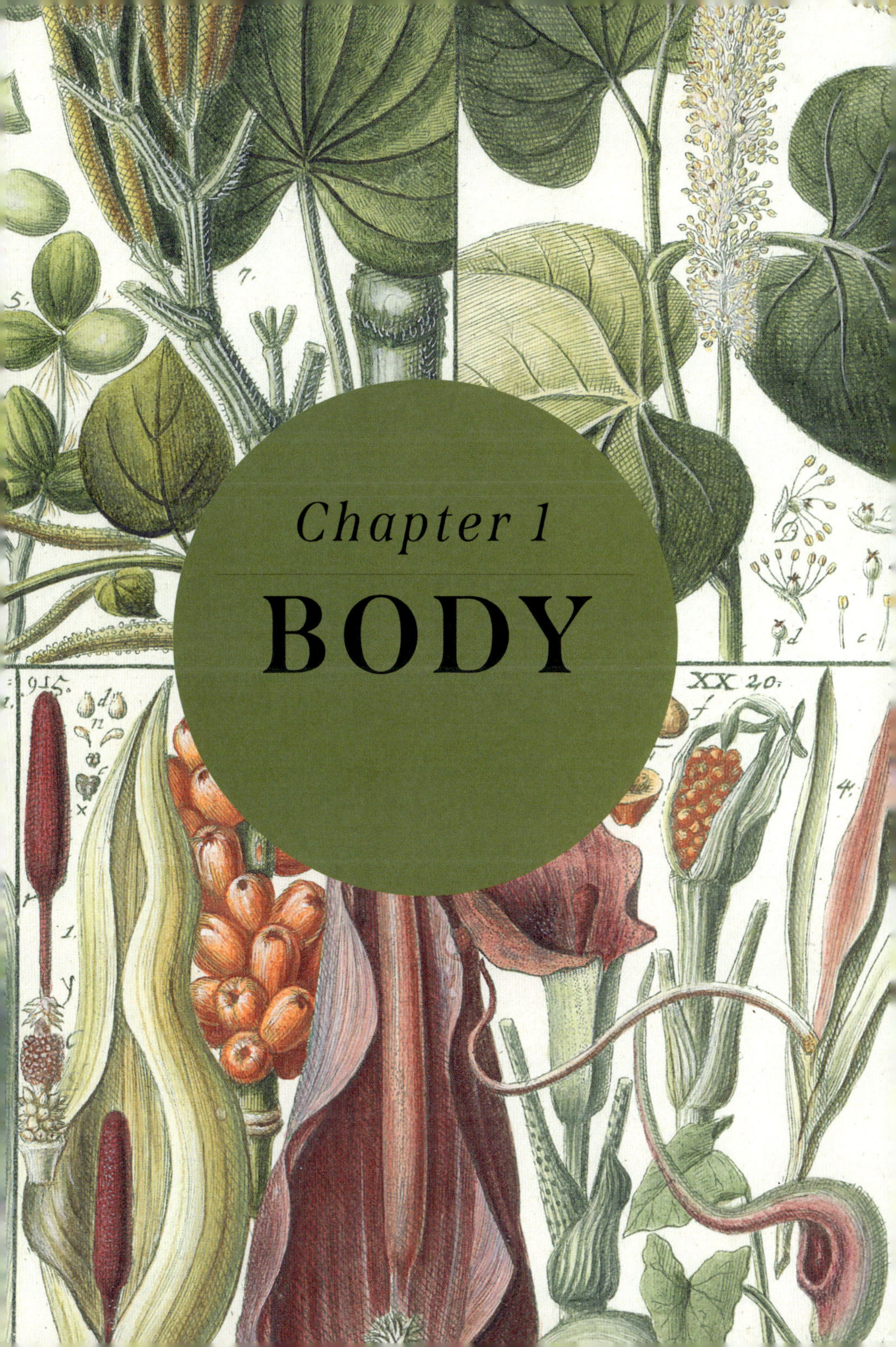

Chapter 1

BODY

Embrace the garden trends that insist less is more

Bad back, how to prevent

There are innumerable jobs in the garden that can cause a bad back. Moving heavy pots. Carrying large branches. Bending over and weeding. In the spring, for the diligent gardener, it can seem that there is no day in which digging is not on the agenda. Certainly, in days past, when 'double digging' was prescribed as the key to planting prep, it was hard toil.

No longer! We live in a 'no-dig' world, except in cases of severe soil compaction. This allows the soil to maintain its structure – and lets the worms get on with it – and means less back-breaking digging for humans. There is even better news, however, because 'no dig' is just the start of what can only be called the 'less is more' gardening revolution.

Reasons for vertebrae to be cheerful include the ubiquitous rewilding or renaturing (a terrible word, but there it is) which involves doing less of almost everything (weeding, bedding, pruning, deadheading). If you do have to dig (and you will, at least a bit), new research using 3D optical tracking shows that the healthy way to go about it is with bent knees (not back) and holding the spade/fork close to the body. Mowing is another source of potential (back) pain but now there are as many ways and times not to mow as to mow and, for some, No Mow May has become No Mow Ever.

We are encouraged to leave perennials over the winter as they provide a habitat which is good for bugs (and backs). Another addition to the 'Not to Do' list is raking up leaves, which are now left for the worms. The natural perennial style of planting is all about embracing plants that last more than a season. Shrubs and trees store carbon which is good for the planet (and backs). We love wildflowers, some of which may have been previously thought of as weeds and therefore required weeding (but no longer). The Japanese have the melodious word *wabi-sabi* for all of this, which is when you find beauty in imperfection and incompleteness. Our backs agree.

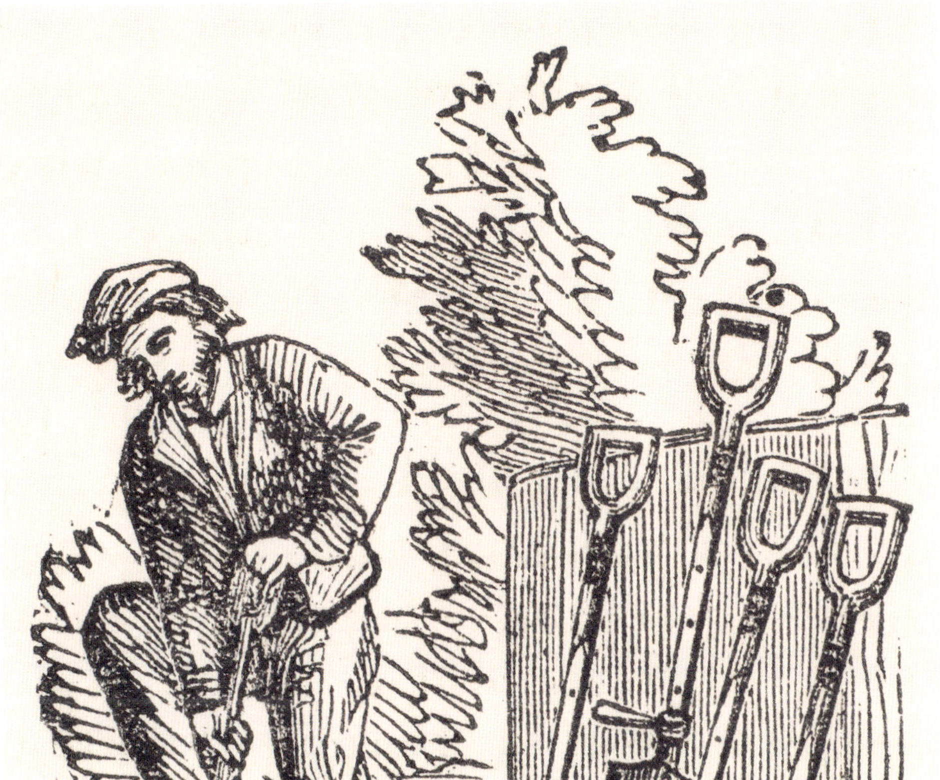

Advertisement for Parkes' Steel Digging Forks & Drilling Tools from *Gardeners' Chronicle & Agricultural Gazette*, 1857.

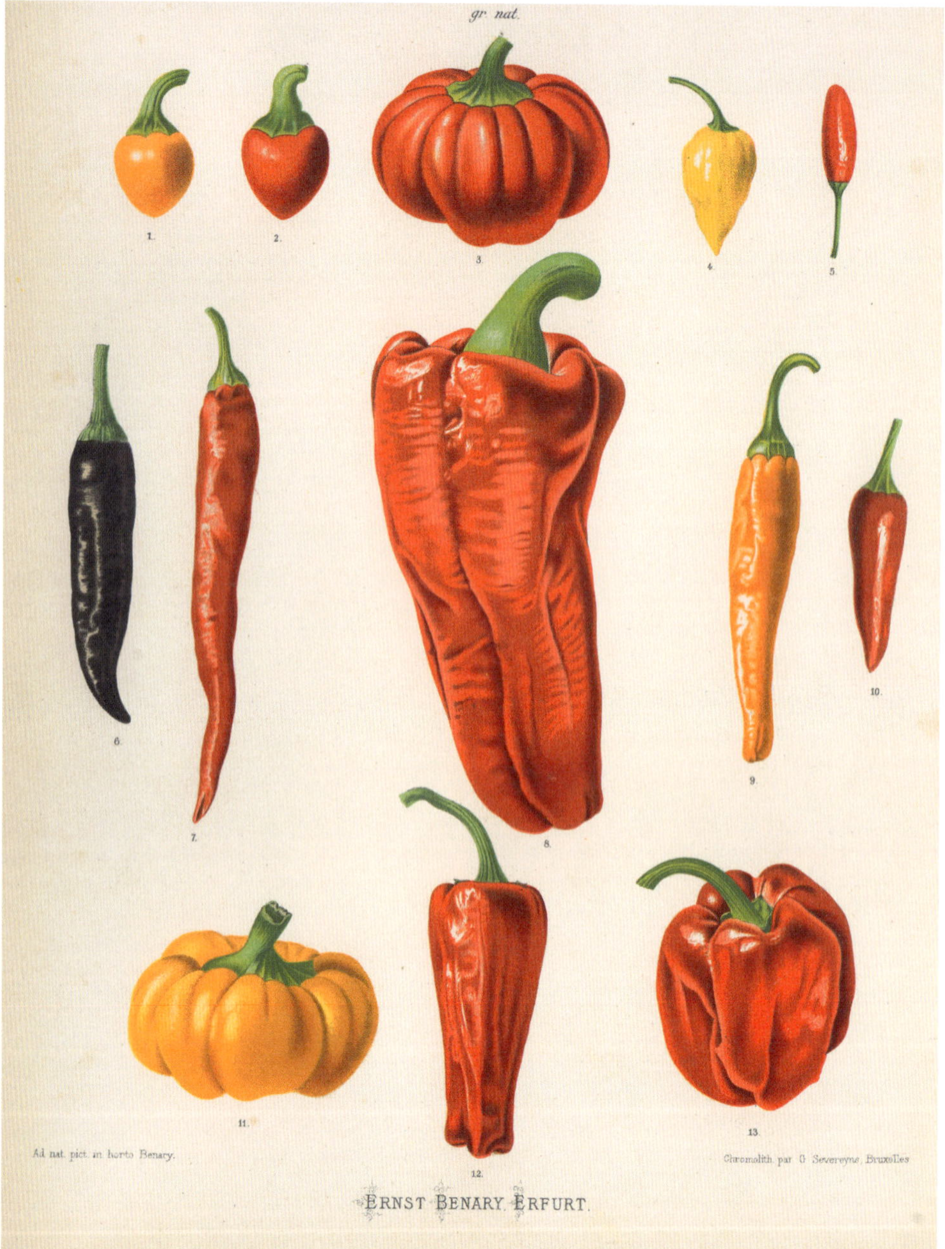

Capsicums by Ernst Benary,
from *Album Benary*, 1877.

Seek out a cream that is red-hot chilli hot

Bad back, aching

The garden may indeed be the cause of your bad back, though less so than in the past (see *Bad Back, How to Prevent*, page 10), but the good news is that it also provides relief as well. Turmeric, ginger and white willow bark are all anti-inflammatory herbs that can reduce pain but, if we go into the greenhouse, we will also find something a little bit spicier. There are thousands of kinds of chilli pepper and, mostly, they are used to enliven food. (In the pre-fridge days, they were helpful because they would slow the growth of microbes, thus making food safer.) But they can also do something rather cool.

When you bite into a chilli, you immediately feel the burn. That is caused by capsaicin, the active ingredient, and when applied to the skin in a cream it can also produce a burning or stinging sensation. But it is also thought that the capsaicin is absorbed by the nerve cells, is transported to the spinal cord, and then decreases the amount of pain-transmitting chemicals sent to the brain. It is a great example of something that is so hot that it is cool.

The capsaicin is applied via cream or patches. The types of peppers used tend to be those with the most available, as in cayenne and serrano peppers (both *Capsicum annuum*), and those highest in capsaicin which include the ghost pepper, aka bhut jolokia, a cultivar of *Capsicum chinense*. It's grown in northeast India and, on the Scoville scale, which is an international gauge of spiciness or heat of chilli peppers, it earns a rating of 1 million. A regular jalapeño is about 2,500 to 8,000 on the scale. So, yes, that's officially hot. You don't have to eat one, though, for your back to feel better.

Willows, like crocodiles, love a marshy environment

Headache, finding relief from

The ancient Egyptians had a garden cure for most things, although this was often combined with an impressive number of other items, some of which now seem extraordinary. Medical papyri, which date from 1550 BCE, call for cures that include eel heads, warmed frogs, ebony shavings, semen, bat blood and multiple sorts of dung. The different papyri, which are rather unfairly named after various Europeans who bought them and had them translated in the 1800s, leave no doubt that the ancient world suffered as we do from headaches of all intensities, including migraines which were referred to as 'pain in half the head'.

The *Ebers Papyrus* set out a cure for headache as follows: mix a peeled onion, fruit of the am tree, salt, setseft [possibly sesame] seeds, honey and abra ointment with cooked swordfish bones, cooked redfish and a cooked crayfish skull. This is to be applied to the head for four days. Another cure, from another papyrus (named after Chester Beatty V), involves a clay crocodile with its mouth stuffed with grain and a linen strip that has the images of at least eight gods attached to the head. Crocodiles were seen as distinctly good things, being divine helpers against evil.

Would you prefer the crayfish or crocodile cure? Or perhaps something else entirely. This can be found in other pieces of papyrus – as well as our gardens today – and that is willow bark. It's not entirely clear what the ancient Egyptians were using it for, though the heart and nervous system seem to be involved, as well as possibly an inflamed wound. In folklore, willow bark seems to have gained quite a following. Greek physician Hippocrates, who lived around 400 BCE, was said to be a fan and various folk cures have credited willow bark with both anti-inflammatory and pain-relieving properties.

So far, so engaging, if relatively unsourced. Fast forward a few thousand years to Chipping Norton in Oxfordshire, England, in 1763, to find the first published account of its medical uses when the Reverend Edward Stone used willow bark extract to treat malarial fever, common in England at the time. Stone believed in the Doctrine of Signatures, which maintained that

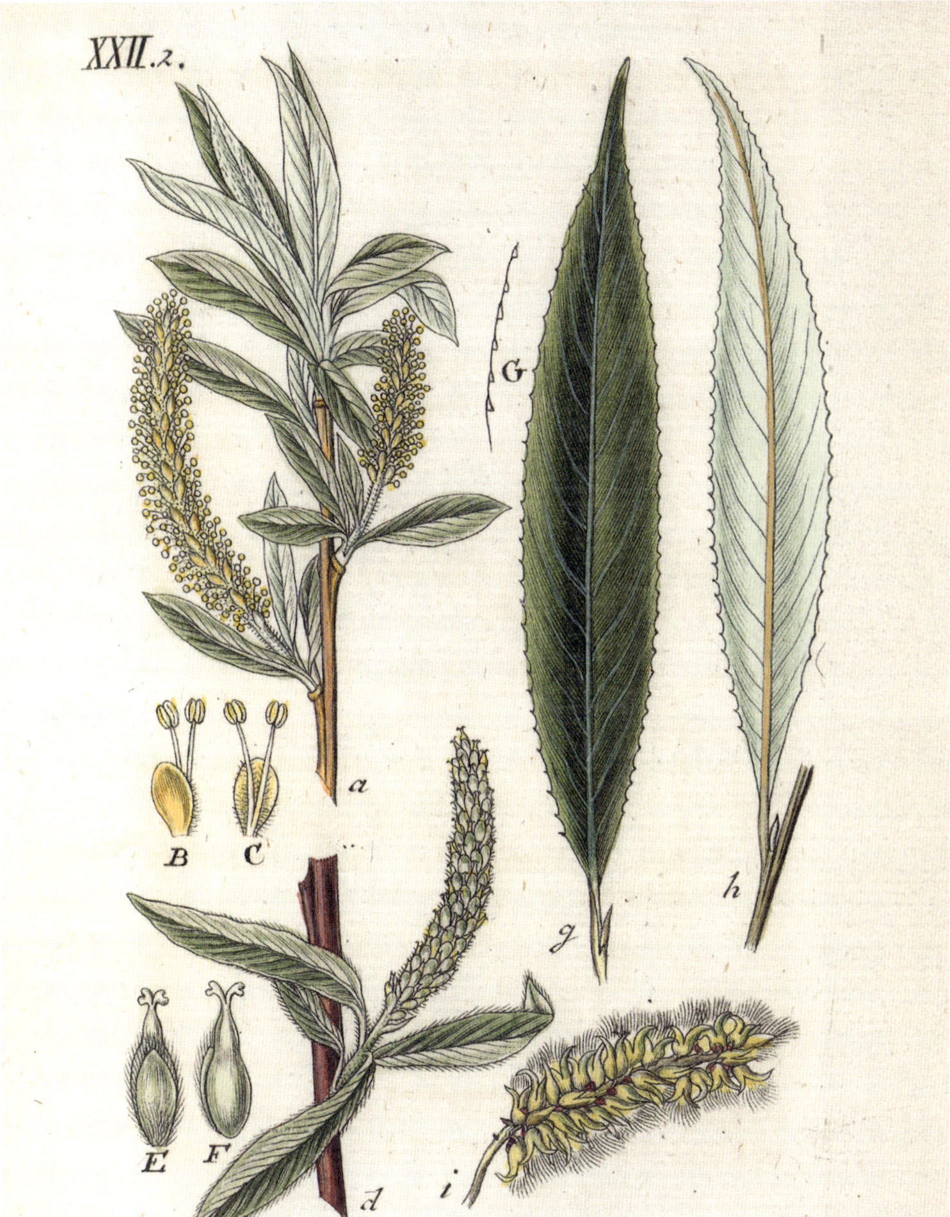

White willow (*Salix alba*) by Jacob Sturm, from *Deutschlands Flora in Abbildungen nach der Natur mit Beschreibungen*, 1801.

cures could often be found close to the source of the malady. His thinking was that willow trees loved a marshy and moist environment and so did fever. (So, of course, do crocodiles, though that is not related at all.)

The Reverend Stone nibbled on a willow twig and was impressed by its bitterness (he knew quinine, a malarial cure, was bitter). He made a powder and was astonished by the results: 'There is the bark of an Englifh tree, which I have found by experience to be a powerful aftringent, and very efficacious in curing aguifh and intermitting diforders.' It would take many more years, and scientists, to turn that discovery into what we know as aspirin. In 1828, scientists isolated what we now recognize as salicin, named after the botanical name of the willow, *Salix alba vulgaris*. (Other species of willow with a high salicin content are also used.) This was later converted in the laboratory to salicylic acid, which was more effective, and then a way was found to reduce its bitterness. It was sold for the first time as aspirin in 1899 by the German company Bayer. It's still in everyday use today, no crocodile required.

'In folklore, willow bark seems to have gained quite a following.'

Get outside in the garden to burn off some calories

Exercise, need to do

Do you feel guilty if you find yourself in the garden instead of the gym? If so, you can stop that thought immediately. As it happens, the garden *is* a gym, just a very nice green one without lots of shiny machines and blaring music. Gardening is all about movement: bending down and back up (use your knees), walking here and there (usually carrying something that weighs a few pounds), using a spade or fork. You'll get toned arms from pruning a hedge, especially if it's a high one, and lots of stretching besides.

Gardening for 30 minutes burns 167 calories (calculated for a person who weighs 70kg/154lb), which is equivalent to playing badminton and more than yoga or gymnastics (149 calories). If you are digging (see *Bad Back*, pages 10 and 13), it's 186 calories, which is the same amount as a brisk walk. You'll burn 298 calories with 30 minutes of running or cycling, but the great thing about gardening, in comparison, is that you are boosting muscle strength and flexibility at the same time. Plus you get to smell the flowers. (For another compelling reason to use your green gym, see *Dementia, Preventing*, page 107.)

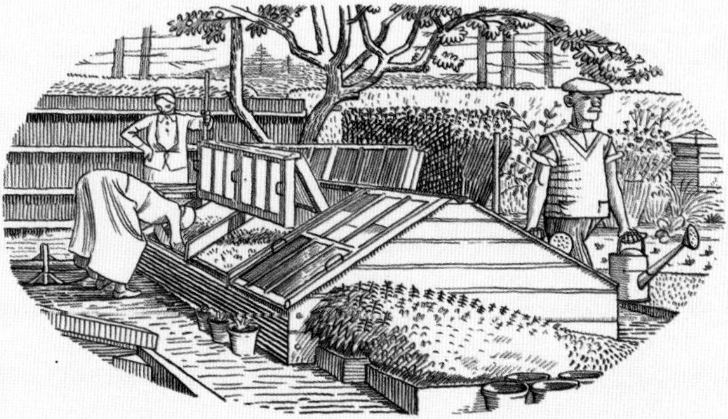

Pen and ink illustration by
Evelyn Mary Dunbar, 1937.

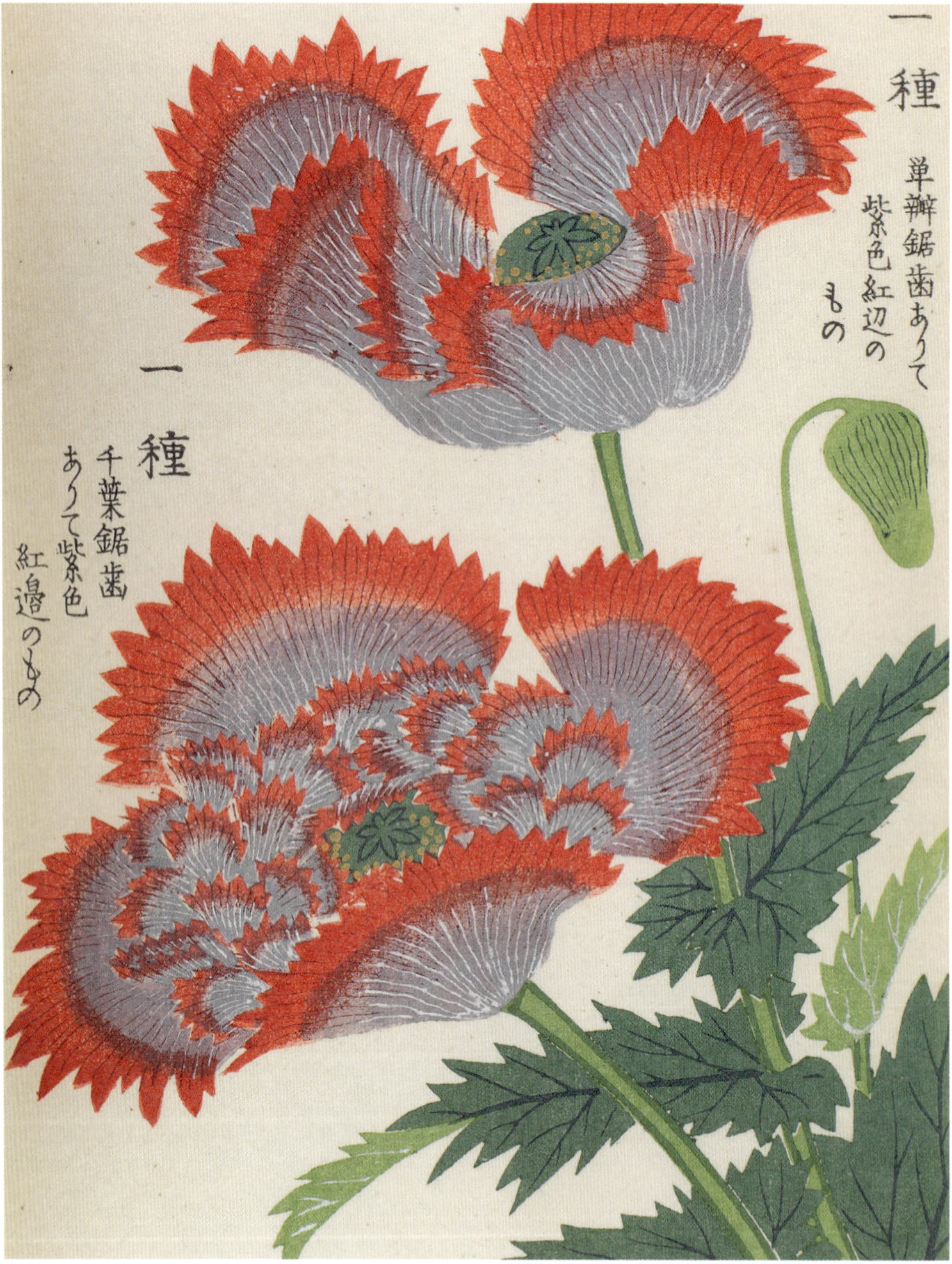

Opium poppy (*Papaver somniferum*) by Iwasaki Tsunemasa, from *Honzō Zufu*, first printed *c.*1830–1844 (second edition, *c.*1920).

Two kinds of poppies served soldiers in the First World War

Pain, relief of

The stories behind two poppies – the corn poppy (*Papaver rhoeas)* and the opium poppy (*P. somniferum*) – converged in a way that will link them forever to the First World War. The 'milk of the poppy', the whitish sap that oozes from the unripe seedheads of *P. somniferum* when they are cut, had long been used medicinally for the relief of extreme pain as well as illicitly on a global scale. There is evidence of humans using opium dating back to 5000 BCE and cultivation is thought to have started in 3400 BCE in Mesopotamia. The sap contains morphine, codeine and thebaine. The first is used to alleviate moderate to extreme pain and the second is a milder pain reliever and cough suppressant. Thebaine is used to make pharmaceutical opioids such as oxycodone. The opium poppy is both the source of an essential medicine that has helped countless people and an illegal drug that has created war, addiction and mayhem in the world. In the plant world, its seedhead is both superhero and super-villain, although it's only its use by us that makes it so.

There is nothing villainous about the corn poppy, or field poppy, though. Its flowers have been used as a mild painkiller for the likes of earache and as a cough medicine. Both poppies are fanatical self-seeders and can pop up in a garden without prior notice. The corn poppy is shorter, growing to less than a metre, with bright scarlet, bowl-shaped flowers. The opium poppy grows up to 1.2m (4ft) and has wide open flowers with large petals and dark purple or yellow stamens. It is not illegal to grow them in the UK (just try and stop them self-seeding), but it is illegal to process them in any way.

In the First World War, opium in the form of morphine was used to treat many of the vast number of soldiers, estimated at 23 million, who were wounded. Medics administered it by needle and, in some cases, the soldiers administered it themselves from a small metal tin that contained phials of morphine. In the churned-up fields, in Belgium and northern France, corn poppies sprang up, creating seas of red that now remain a symbol of remembrance. 'In Flanders fields, the poppies blow/Between the crosses, row on row,' begins a poem by the Canadian doctor and First World War soldier Lt-Col John McCrae who would have known both types of poppies well.

The hills are alive with a remedy for your ills

Bruising and muscle aches, how to soothe

Here's a cure that you can yodel about. Arnica is a bright yellow, daisy-like flower that grows in alpine meadows. Legend has it that its healing properties were first noticed by German goatherders as they watched their charges eat the flowers after they were injured. That seems unlikely, but what is undisputed is that *Arnica montana* has been used for centuries by Europeans (and Native Americans) to treat muscle aches and bruising, with creams or as a poultice made by diluting the flowers in water. Clinical studies have had mixed results, though research in the 1980s did show that arnica contains helenalin which has anti-inflammatory and mild pain-killing properties. Inconclusive studies have had absolutely no effect on its huge popularity, however, and it has been over-foraged in the wild to the extent that it has had to be protected in many countries, including Germany. That will please the goats at least.

'Arnica's healing properties were first noticed by German goatherders as they watched their charges eat the flowers after they were injured.'

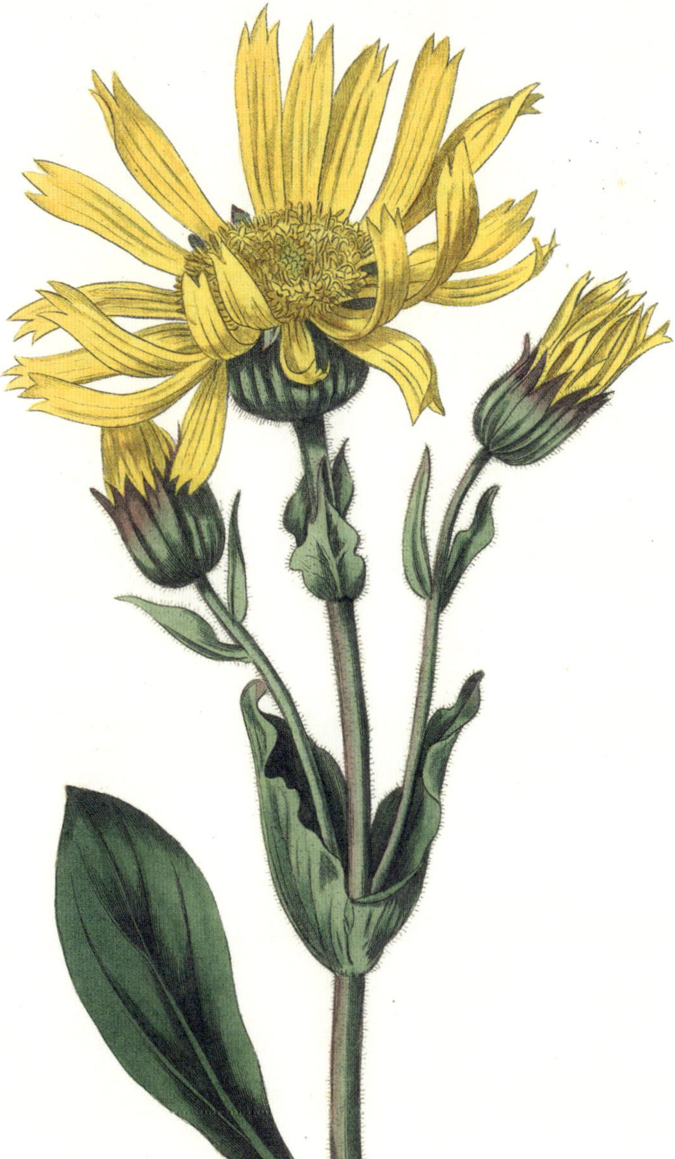

Arnica montana, illustration published in *Curtis's Botanical Magazine*, 1815.

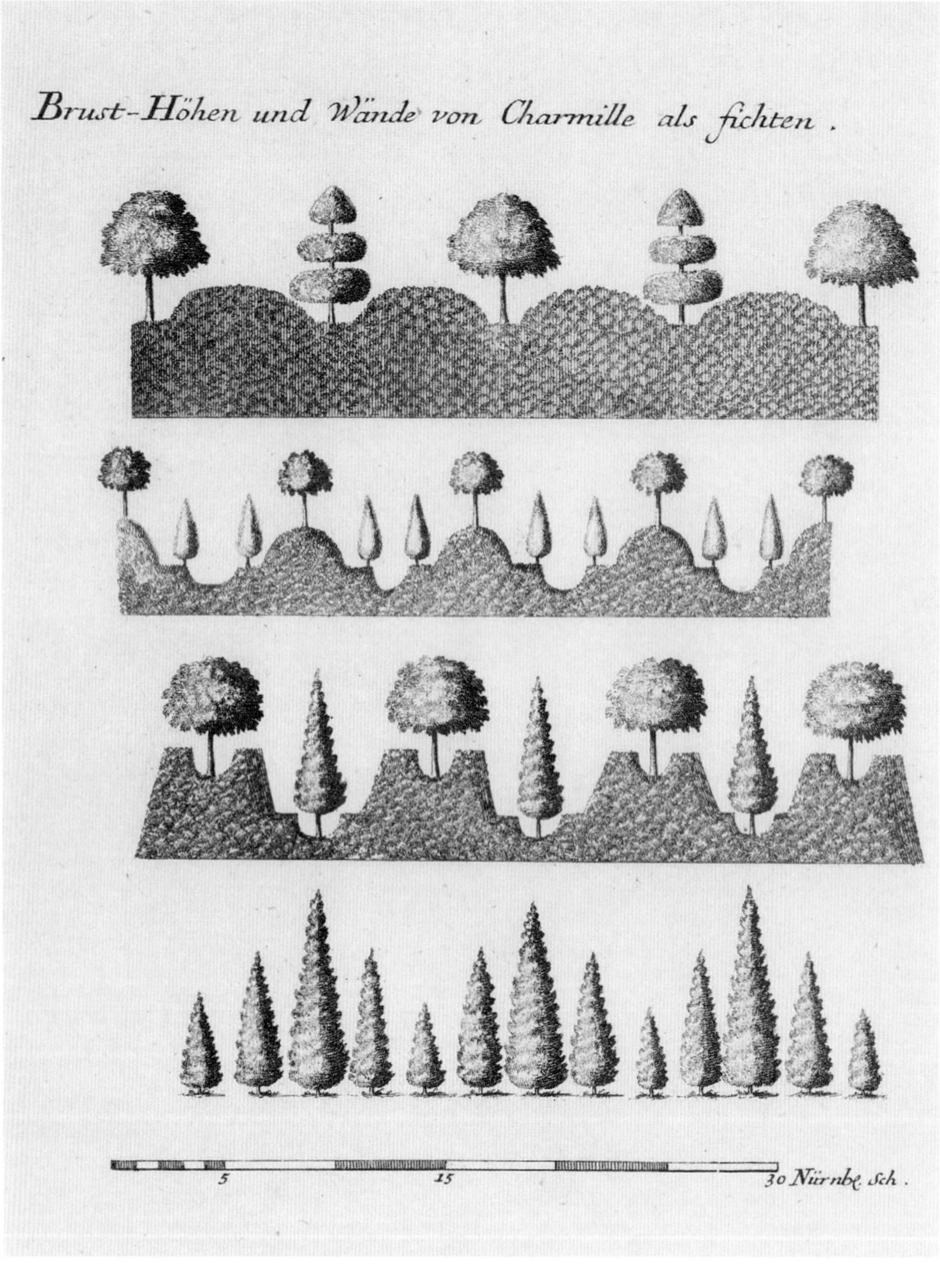

'Blobby' hedgerow styles: Johann David Fülck, from *Neue Garten Lust, oder Völliges Ornament*, 1710–20.

You feel you are a blob with no get up and go

Energy, lack of

There is no doubt that being a blob or blobby is not something to aspire to. For starters, there has been a lack of positive blob role models. There is the unappetizing slime mould *Physarum polycephalum*, for instance. In computing, a BLOB is a Binary Large Object. In Hollywood, *The Blob* is a 1958 horror sci-fi movie with an ameboid alien who crashes to Earth and tries to absorb mankind. You see the problem. No one wants to be any of these things.

Thankfully, gardening does not care about such simplistic stereotypes. We know that a blob can be a thing of beauty. Some may define a blob as a 'shapeless mass', but we know that it is a ball that is slightly squashed and so is pruned to be wider than it is tall. If you feel that you are becoming a blob (and not in a good way), get out in the garden and get pruning.

Making a blob is not for the lackadaisical. You can have a solo blob or create a group (a blobbery) of three or more. Blobs are all about creating year-round structure in your garden. Most blobs are evergreen shrubs that, on their own, may not be seen as the most exciting but, as a group or in contrast to other plants, can become a shrubscape of undulating mounds that can be separate or knitted together, with varying leaf textures, flowering times and seasonal colour.

A key trait of blob plants is that unblobbed, they are rather ordinary. Think cotoneasters, the Portuguese laurel (or *Prunus lusitanica* 'Myrtifolia'), *Viburnum tinus*, silverberry (*Shepherdia argentea*), honeysuckle (*Lonicera*). The transformation is in the pruning: turn over your shears, so they are slightly domed, and clip the plant two to four times a year (depending on growth), ensuring it is wider than it is tall. It makes sense to mix fast growers (honeysuckle) with slow (yew). You can also experiment with the shape, creating a blob dome, for instance, by removing lower branches. Blobs look great when contrasted with flowering grasses or with topiary triangles or, even, a cloud-pruned shrub. Blobs are not about feeling bad but rather being brave, bold and experimental.

Your sex life is uninspiring and lacks that certain something

Drab sex life, spicing up

If your sex life has taken a turn for the worse, then take a few lessons from the not-so-humble frog, as seen in gardens galore. Amphibian sex is, well, just a bit wild. They don't call it the Kermit Sutra for nothing. It all begins by early spring when a male frog makes it clear he is bored bored BORED with hibernating. He knows what he wants and he heads for 'his' pond with a plan. 'Sex! Sex! Sex!' he cries in his low, croaking call (translation accurate).

Here's how it works. He's the showboater. She's the choosy one. Frog experts say that what female frogs find sexy varies around the world. Some females like complex calls, others prefer the deepest or loudest. The male just keeps on calling. He's keen and believes that 'Sex! Sex! Sex!' is going to work in the end. Plus, it's all he knows.

Frog sex is called 'amplexus', which is a fancy word for what might be called a 'love hug' or (sigh) 'cuddle'. The male frog, which is slightly smaller than the female, climbs onto her back and grasps her behind the forelegs or around the 'waist'. His hold is pretty good, as the grip of his toes and nuptial pads improves during the mating season. Besides the basic piggyback position, there are variations in amplexus, including the 'dorsal straddle', 'head straddle' and one called 'independent' which is tail to tail. There is also one called 'glued', which is a good description of most frog sex because they can stay in amplexus for days.

A popular pond can quickly descend into orgiastic scenes. Couples bob up and down, hang out just below the surface, overlap with other couples. They do not seem to be doing much, heads facing forward, lips closed. At some point, the female expels her eggs and the male reacts simultaneously, sending out the sperm to fertilize. Soon more frogs are coupling amid the frogspawn. Frog sex is all done externally, but they clearly like to have quite a bit of skin-on-skin action. What are the lessons of frog sex? Don't be shy. Be consensual. Be patient. Be sexy. For days.

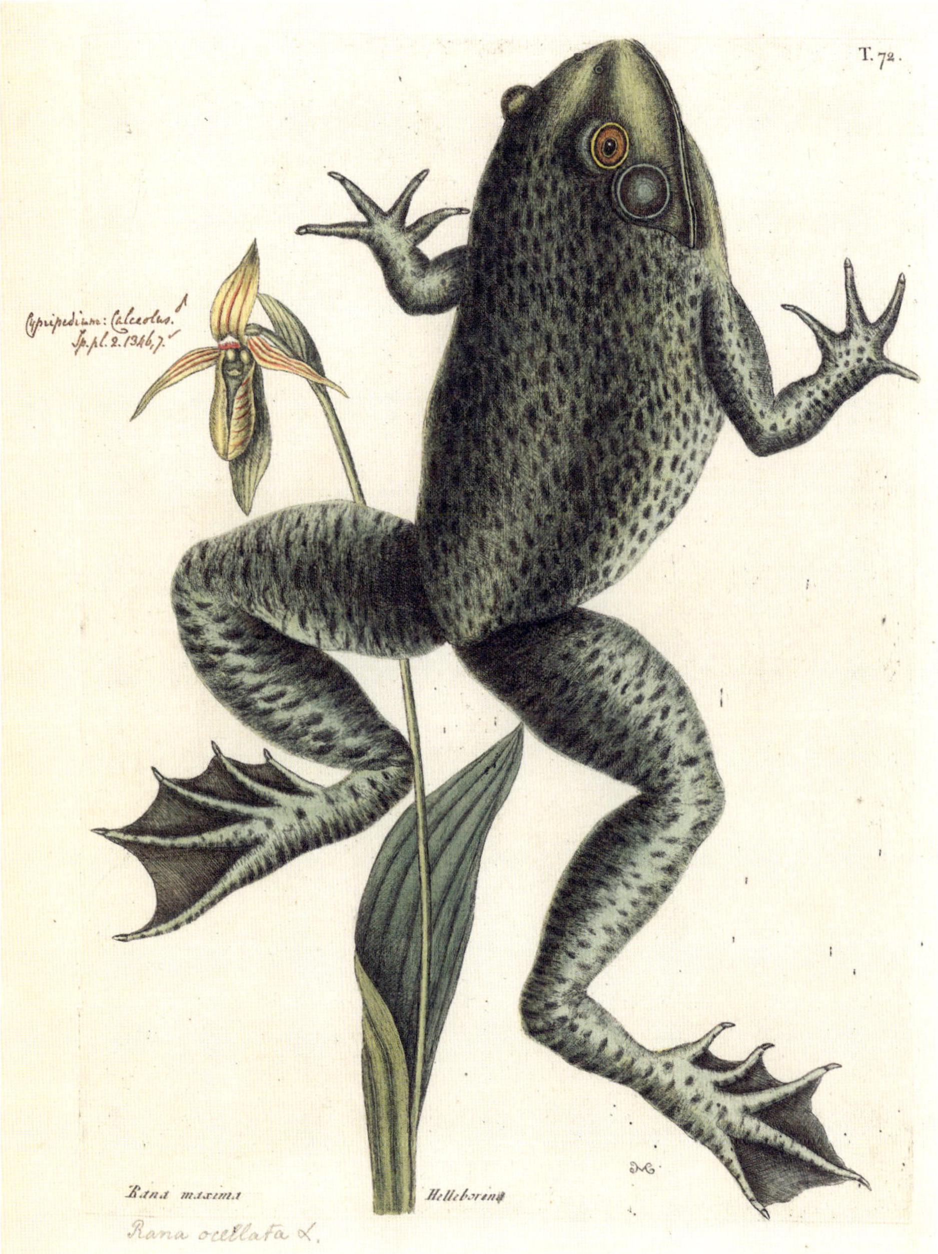

Bull frog (*Rana maxima*) by Mark Catesby, from *The Natural History of Carolina, Florida and the Bahama Islands*, 1754.

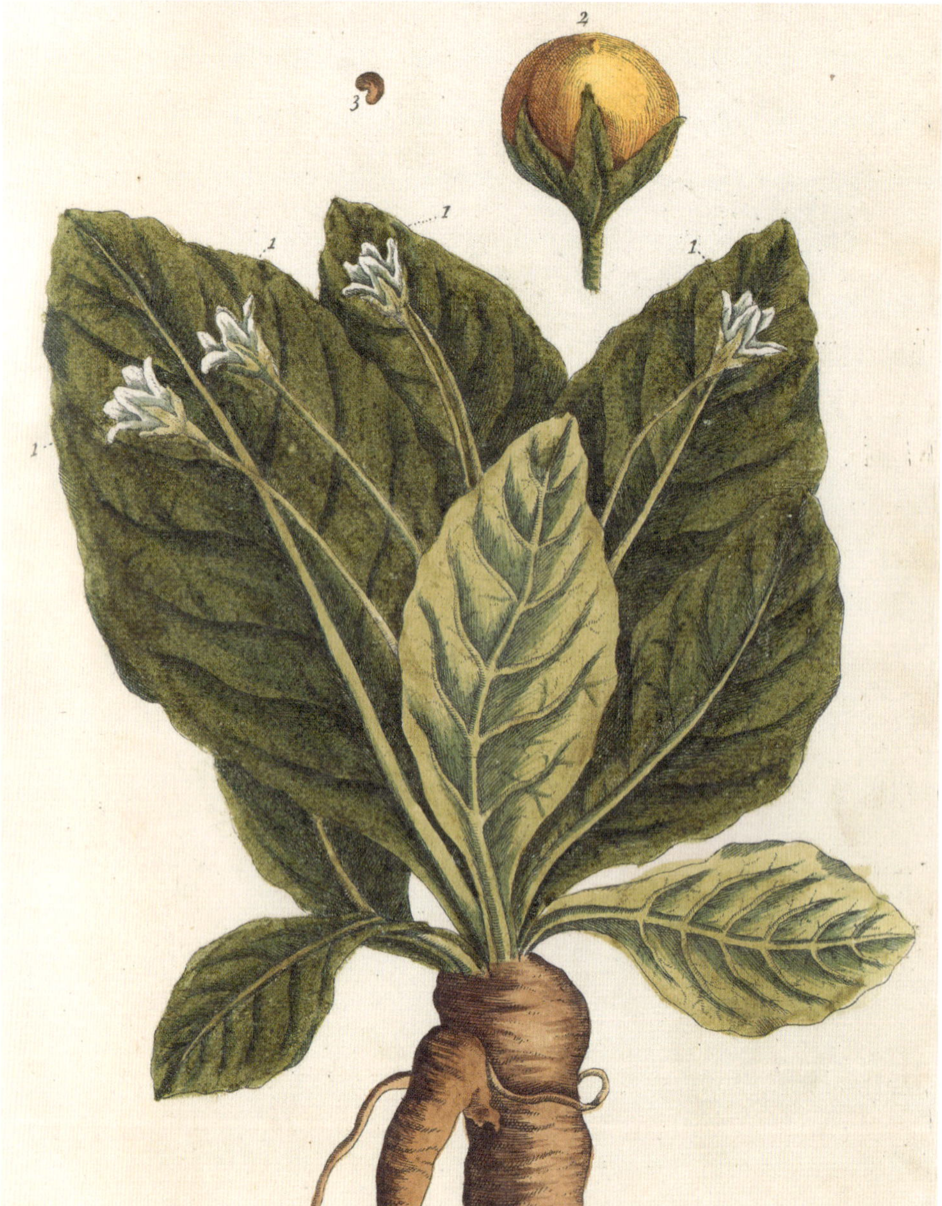

Mandrake by Elizabeth Blackwell,
from *A Curious Herbal*, Vol. 2, 1737–39.

There is no lack of advice from ancient folklore

Pregnant, desire to be

There are so many folkloric garden cures for women when it comes to getting pregnant that it seemed a shame to pick just one. Of course, no one knows if any of them, or indeed all of them, will work, but there are enough here to offer a planting plan for an 'I Want To Get Pregnant' flower bed. This is what you could do if you want to plant a seed:

- Pick St John's wort (*Hypericum perforatum*): The idea is to get naked and walk somewhere (hopefully not too urban) to pick some St John's wort. You will be pregnant within a year. (Please note that you only need to *pick* the plant. Anything else – including infusing or eating – is not advised.)
- Plant parsley (*Petroselinum crispum*): It's not the easiest thing to get parsley to sprout and, in general in the past, the cause of this problem was seen to be the Devil himself. It is said that women should avoid planting (or buying) it unless they want to get pregnant. Indeed, virgins are advised to avoid planting it completely.
- Dance around a silver birch (*Betula pendula*): A special tree to the Druids who saw it as the goddess tree. Best results expected if danced around as a living maypole.
- Make tea from raspberry (*Rubus idaeus*) leaves, sometimes known as 'the women's herb'. A strong tea was said to prepare the womb for pregnancy and can be drunk before a marriage ceremony.
- Wear mugwort (*Artemisia vulgaris*): Witches' herb, long seen to promote fertility, especially in cases of spiritual stagnation. Can be burned as incense during fertility rites or worn in sachets around the waist.
- Sleep with a mandrake (*Mandragora officinarum*): Go to sleep with a mandrake root under your pillow. This is all about its forked roots, which often look like a person. The advice is to find a mandrake root that looks more female than male (see *Impregnate, Desire To...*, page 28) but please note that mandrake should come with a giant warning sticker as it has hallucinatory, narcotic and sedative side effects and is not to be trifled with.

For men, it's all geared towards performance

Impregnate, desire to

There is almost as much advice for men as for women when it comes to wanting to have a child. But for men, the advice is all about sperm and being able to deliver them. Here are a few top tips on how to become more virile:

- Walnuts (*Juglans regia*): A study from the University of California (L.A.) School of Nursing found eating 75g (2½oz) of walnuts daily improved sperm vitality, motility and morphology. It's not known why, though walnuts contain antioxidants, micronutrients and alpha-linolenic acid (an essential fatty acid). You'll need to find a mature walnut tree if you don't want to wait years, as walnut trees grow very, very slowly.
- Horny goat weed (*Epimedium*), aka the herbal Viagra: This evergreen perennial that gardeners know as epimediums has been used for centuries in Chinese medicine to boost male fertility. The legend goes that a goatherder saw that his charges became unusually amorous after eating it. But please note, modern studies are limited and inconclusive.
- Sow wild oats: The phrase 'sowing his wild oats' usually referred to a young man who was having too much fun before settling down. But there is also a folklore belief that wild oats (*Avenua fatua*) themselves can get in on the act, as they are rumoured to be a testosterone enhancer.
- Mandrake (*Mandragora officinarum*): This is the mother (or father) lode when it comes to herbal folklore and fertility (see *Pregnant, Desire to Be,* page 27). For thousands of years, it was believed that the root should be put under your pillow or worn on the body and in charms to promote potency. But nothing about the mandrake is easy and even acquiring it was fraught with difficulty, including, apparently, death. The plant, which is a narcotic, hallucinogenic and sedative, was said to emit a hugely powerful cry when uprooted, a wail so powerful that it could kill. The herbalist solution? Attach the plant to a hungry dog who would race past it (heading for a bowl of food), thus uprooting it. This way, if anyone died, it was the dog and not the herbalist. Not for the faint-hearted.

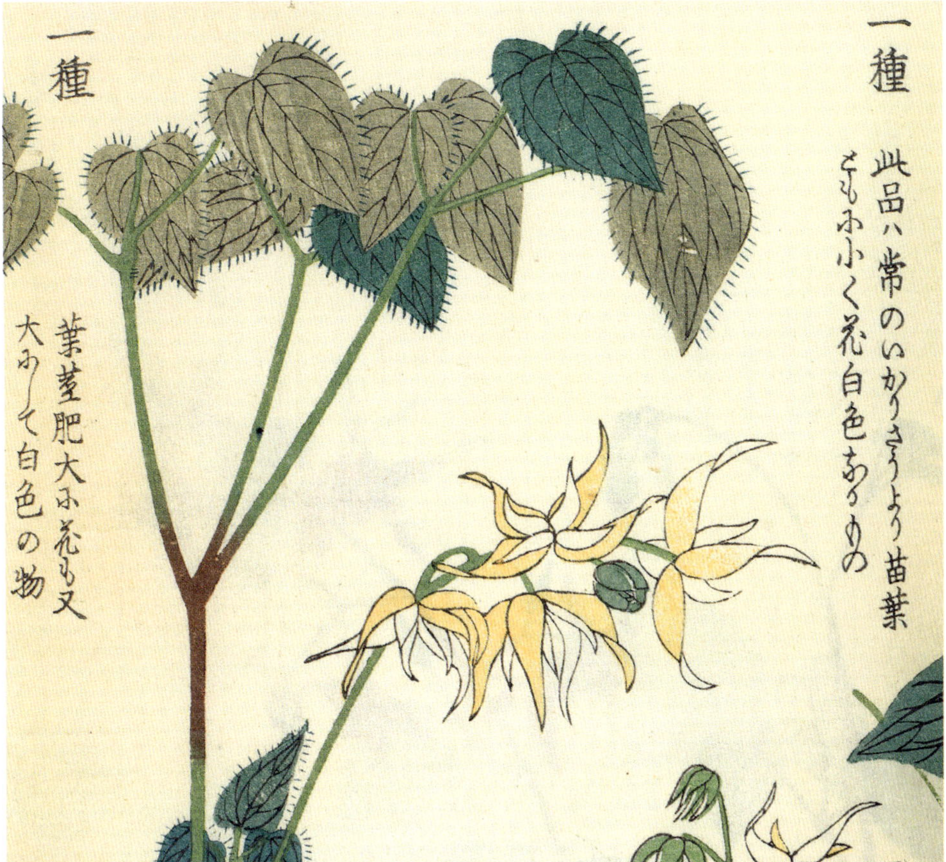

Epimedium by Iwasaki Tsunemasa, from *Honzō Zufu*,
first printed *c.*1830–1844 (second edition, *c.*1920).

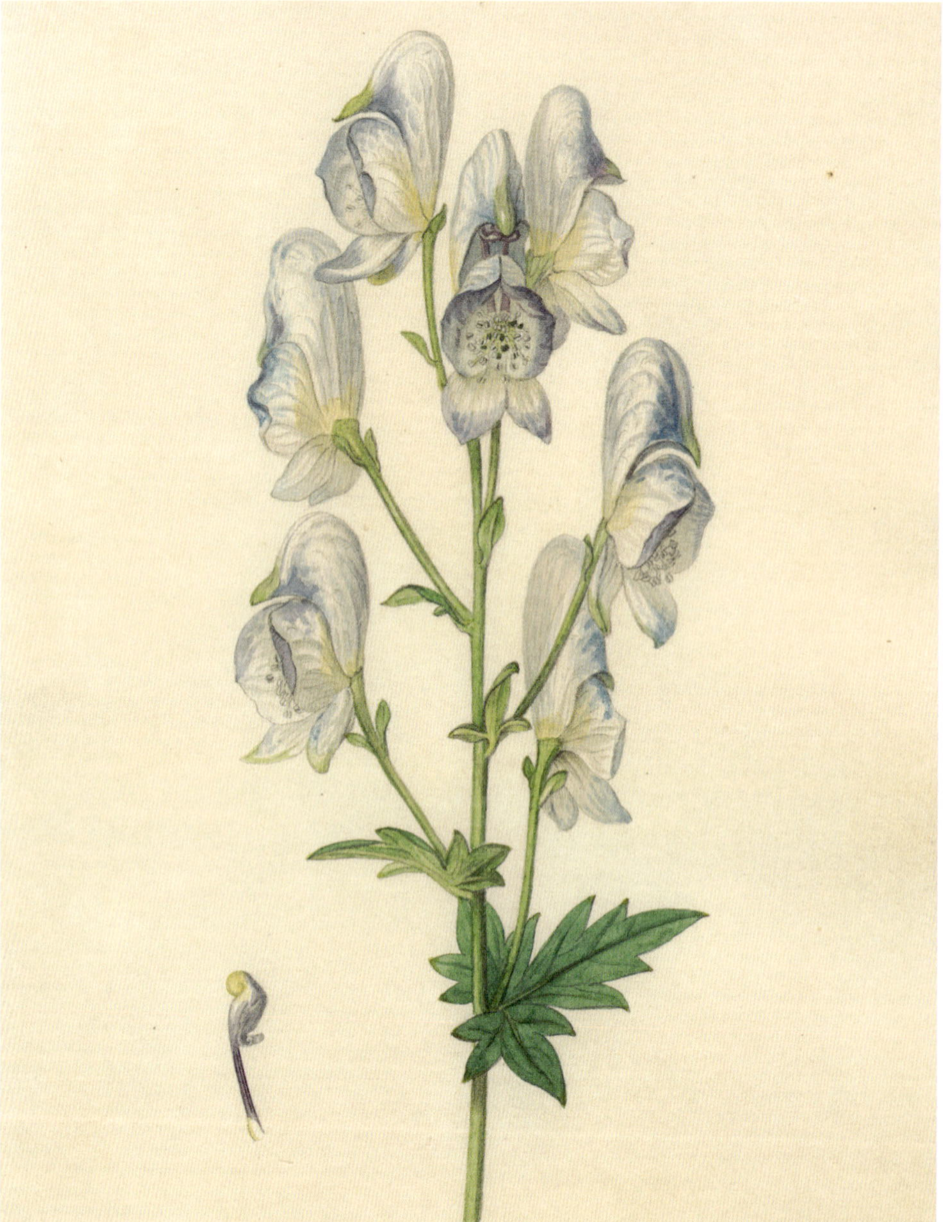

Aconitum variegatum, watercolour on paper by James Sowerby, 1815.

What to do if you are fearful of becoming a werewolf

Howl, desire to

It's a physical thing, the desire to howl. In normal circumstances, if there be such a thing when howling is nigh, this is not in itself alarming. Indeed, as parents of tuneless children know, some singing can be close to howling, though a human howl tends to be a long and rather doleful cry. It's quite different from that of wolves who howl to bond, hunt and just hang out. When in a pack, wolves howl together but not on the same note: the result makes the pack sound larger and is quite melodic in its own way.

If you have a desire to howl – and there is no obvious reason, such as being made redundant or eating a particularly hot chilli – you may fear that you are becoming a werewolf. This is almost surely incorrect as werewolves are fictional beings that are the product of Balkan folklore. Even discounting that, it's not easy to shapeshift from human to wolf, though it can and does happen in Hollywood. The most common way to become a werewolf is to be bitten by one. If you can rule that out, you need to take stock of other factors. Is it night? If so, is there a moon? Is it bright? Even if all those components are in play, as long as it's not mid- or late summer, it is fine. Because that's when the wolf's bane (*Aconitum*) blooms and, as everyone who has seen *The Wolf Man* (1941) knows, that's when everything could start kicking off.

The idea that wolf's bane is involved in turning people into werewolves is another Hollywood fiction because, traditionally, it was seen as an anti-werewolf cure. The plant, which is also known as monk's hood or aconite, is more than a metre tall, with spikes of blue (or sometimes yellow) hood-like flowers. All parts are poisonous to the point where you should use gloves when handling. It was used to poison arrows and spears in ancient times to kill animals (and indeed wolves). In the Middle Ages, the idea that it could cure lycanthropy, which is when someone wants to be a wolf, was floated but often with fatal results. The same problem occurred as an anti-werewolf cure. The basic message here is clear: if you have the desire to howl, feel free, but stay clear of the wolf's bane.

There's a simple cure with a formidable pedigree

Sunburn (or frostbite), how to alleviate

Aloe vera has quite the reputation. The ancient Egyptians called it the 'plant of immortality'. Cleopatra herself reportedly used it in her daily beauty routine. In ancient Greece, it is said that Alexander the Great was advised by his tutor Aristotle to conquer the island of Socotra, in the Arabian Sea, to secure supplies of the plant for his wounded soldiers. *Aloe vera* was reputed to soothe rashes, heal wounds, settle stomachs and act as a laxative or 'cleanser'. Christopher Columbus was a fan, calling aloe an indispensable 'cure'. Mahatma Gandhi credited aloe with helping him fast for longer periods of time. An impressive group of celebrity endorsements.

How true is all of this? You can safely say that *Aloe vera* is, indeed, legendary and it has certainly been used for millennia as a cure for various issues. Whether Cleopatra (or Aristotle) was a devotee is not really known. It certainly did get around. Native to the rugged Hajar Mountains of what is now Oman, it was traded extensively in both the Old World and (starting with Columbus) to the New World. It is sometimes called a cactus but is a succulent, from the lily family, thriving in warm and dry climates in ultra-harsh conditions. The fleshy, pointy leaves have a layer of yellow latex which is responsible for the laxative effect, the use of which has been banned in some countries. They also contain a gel that is mostly water and includes a mix of amino acids, lipids, sterols and vitamins.

It's the gel that concerns us here because if you have sunburn (or indeed frostbite), this will soothe your skin and, as the pain ebbs, your soul. It is rich in antioxidants and is a natural hydrating moisturizer, which also may help with peeling. *Aloe vera* is a regular on the health and beauty shelves and you can buy it in a large range of creams, potions and lotions. Even better, you can grow it yourself, although if you live in a cooler climate, it will have to be as a houseplant. When you need some soothing, simply snap off part of a leaf and ooze the gel onto your skin. It's almost too easy.

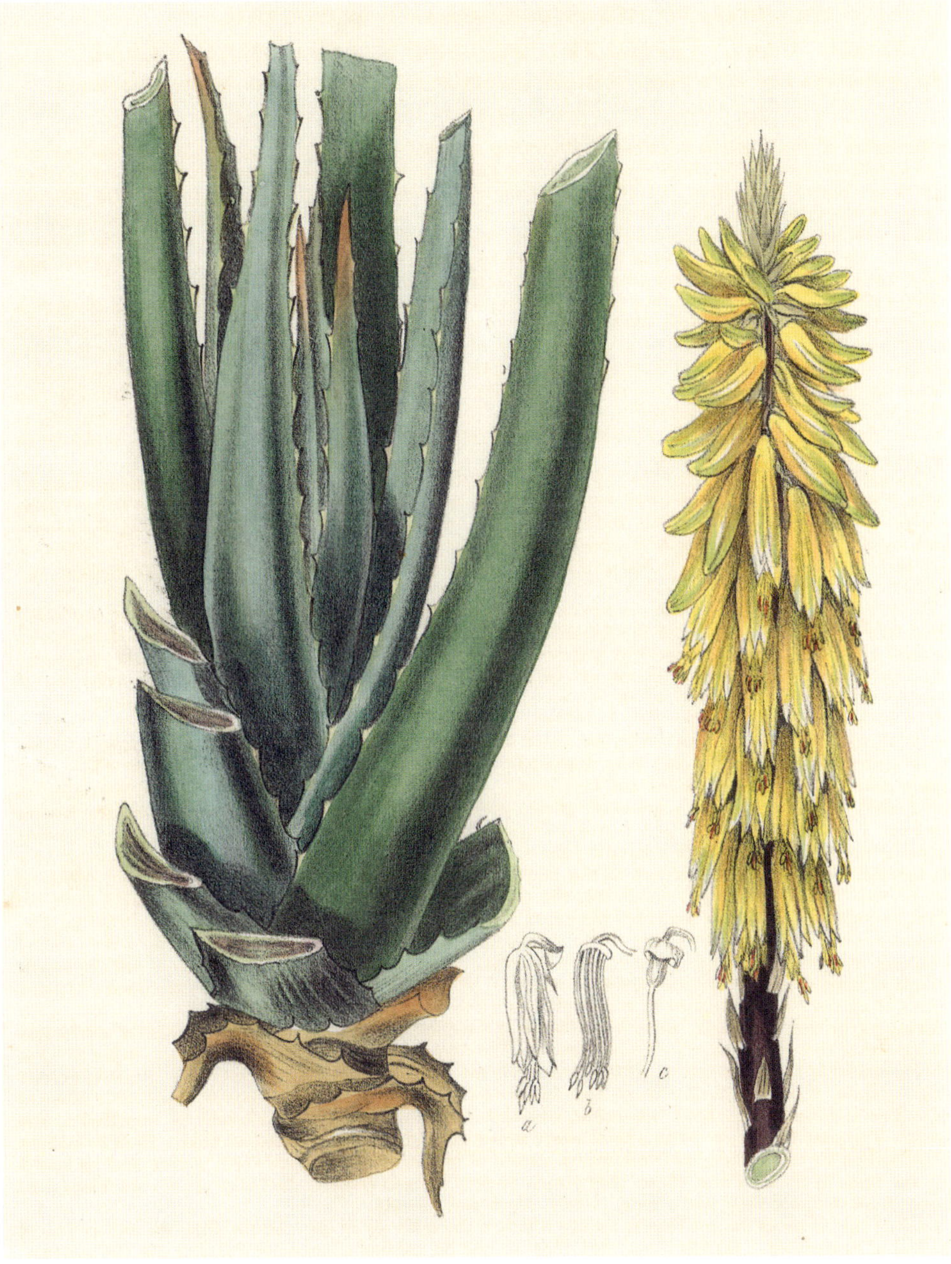

Aloe vera by Mary Ann Burnett, from *Plantae Utiliores, or Illustrations of Useful Plants*, Vol. 4, 1850.

A Wild West story about the greatest cure that ever existed

Snakebite, treating

Roll up, roll up, and hear a story of a medicine so powerful that it can cure everything from serpent bites to cholera. It was the early 1870s during the Wild West era and, smack dab in the middle of the American Midwest, in the small town called Pawnee City in Nebraska, something wild was certainly going on. Dr H C F Meyer, a German immigrant, was sure he had 'discovered' one of the (if not *the*) most powerful cures of all time. It used the root of the native prairie flower *Echinacea angustifolia,* which is also known as purple coneflower and/or snakeroot. Dr Meyer had used it in a herbal concoction that he had patented as 'Meyer's Blood Purifier'. Now he was ready to introduce it to the world.

It may indeed have been the case that echinacea was new to Western medicine, but Dr Meyer would have known full well that he hadn't discovered anything at all. He knew that echinacea roots had been used for centuries by the medicine men and women of the Plains Indians tribes as a remedy for a wide variety of ailments, including coughs, colds, rabies, snakebite, sore throat and toothache. (These, for instance, are the instructions for how the Kiowa and Cheyenne tribes treated colds and sore throats: 'Chew a piece of Echinacea root and let the saliva run down the throat.')

This didn't bother Meyer in the slightest. He was determined that fame and fortune would be his, if only he could convince the medical establishment beyond Pawnee City. He sent his potion (and some root) to prominent doctors, boasting that Meyer's Blood Purifier was a 'slayer of all ailments'. He claimed that it could cure cholera morbus (now known as acute gastroenteritis), sore legs, scrofula, carbuncles, fever, insect stings, syphilis and gonorrhoea, rabies and – perhaps most exciting of all – rattlesnake bites. In 600 cases of snakebite and other ailments, he said, his amazing blood purifier had never once failed to cure. Such was Dr Meyer's zeal that he offered to travel the 1,120km (700 miles) to Cincinnati, with his own rattlesnakes if none could be conjured up there, to let himself be bitten 'freely' in front of medical authorities. He would then cure himself only with his blood purifier. The doctors turned him down, which was lucky for him.

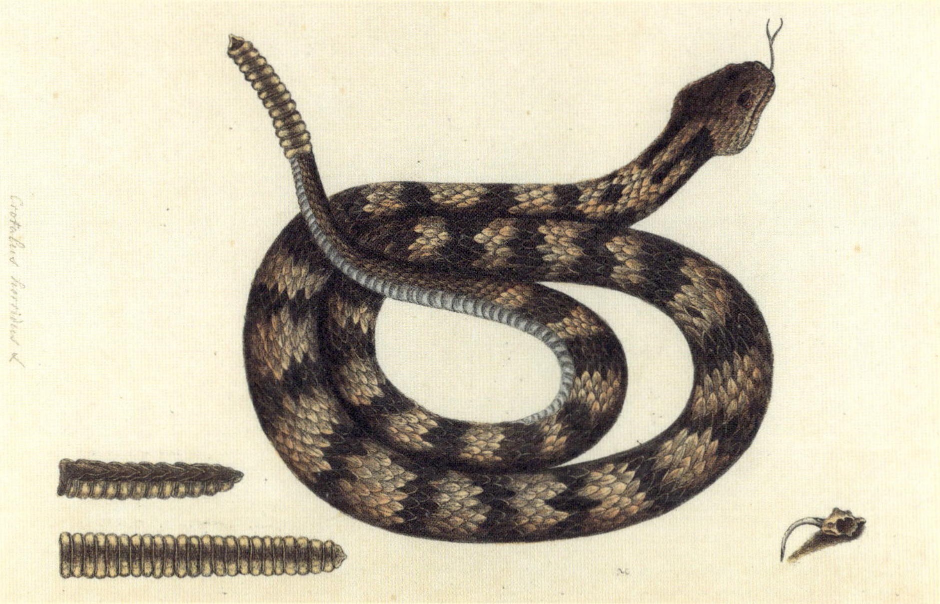

Timber rattlesnake (*Vipera caudisona*) by Mark Catesby, from *The Natural History of Carolina, Florida and the Bahama Islands*, 1754.

Dr Meyer wasn't alone, of course, as this was the era of fake miracle cures when the likes of useless but harmless sarsaparilla (made from the root of *Smilax officinalis*, alcohol and herbals) were sold by travelling salesmen who knew how to tell an outlandishly tall tale. There was one prominent doctor who did test Dr Meyer's root, though, and found that for his wife, who had cancer, it offered some relief and, indeed, more than any other remedy. It wasn't a cure (she did die), but her testimony meant it had been introduced to the medical world and that was all the encouragement Dr Meyer needed. He was reportedly off and running, selling his miracle cure, brandishing his rattlesnake stories, to any and all customers.

Meyer may have been as slippery as a snake, but he was in tune with his times – a Wild West chancer with a stolen cure and a desire for fame and fortune. Echinacea today is a popular herbal remedy, particularly for colds, but clinical results are mixed. If you do get bitten by a rattlesnake, don't head to the garden to dig up your purple coneflower. The only cure for venomous snakes is to be injected with an anti-venom. Go to hospital – pronto.

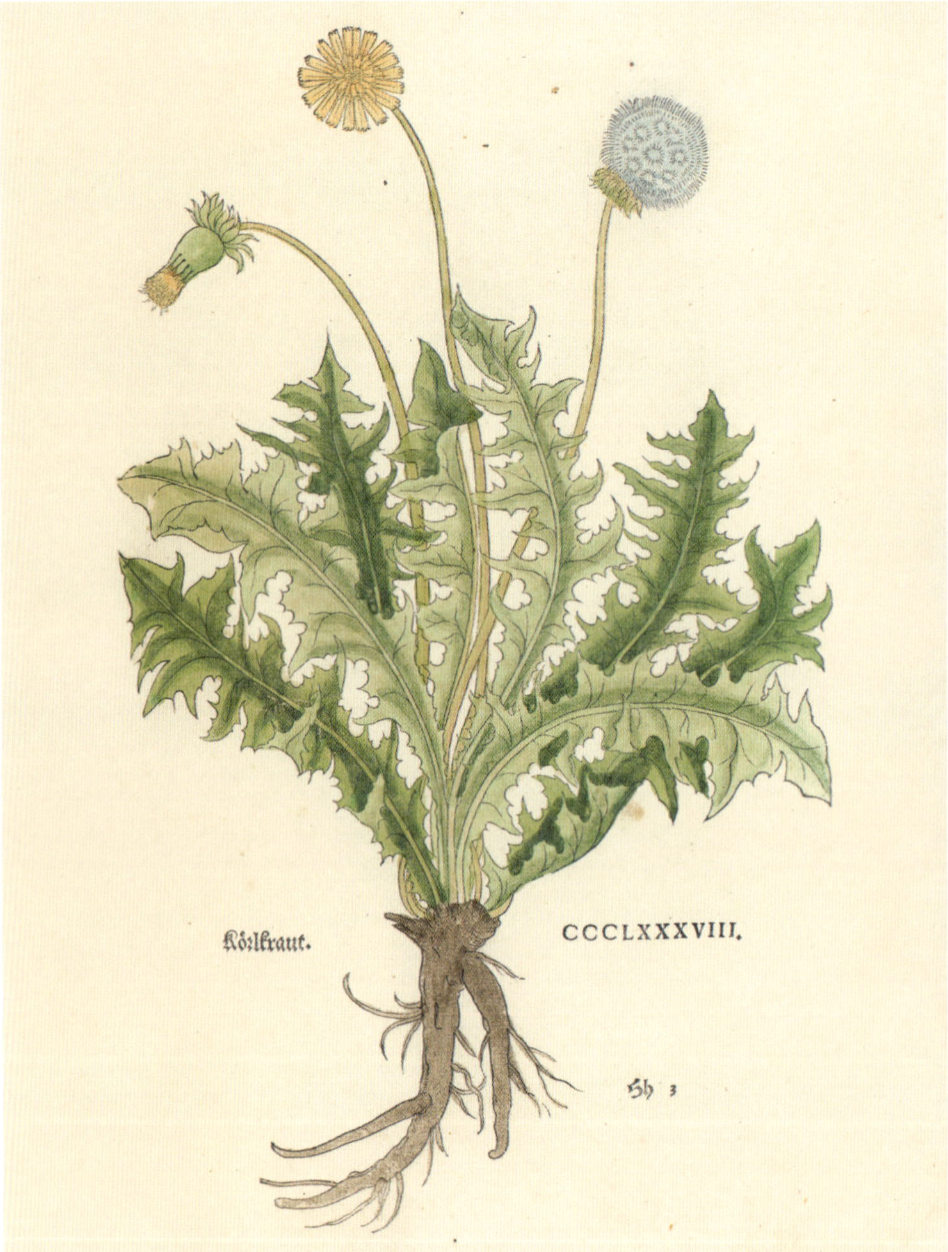

Dandelion (*Taraxacum officinale*) by Leonhart Fuchs, from *De historia stirpium commentarii insignes...*, 1542.

There's a superweed out there that knows what to do

Bloating and constipation, relief from

Dandelions are one of those plants that appears indestructible. They grow everywhere and anywhere and, as Nicholas Culpeper noted in his *Complete Herbal* of 1653: 'It flowereth in one place or another almost all year long.' Its long taproot is the bane of lawn-lovers everywhere and its seed clocks are incredibly efficient at dispersing their 150 to 200 seeds. Bees love them and children delight in puffing away at the seedheads (the number of seeds left will tell you what time it is in fairyland). Gardeners are divided into those who embrace *Taraxacum officinale* as a wildlife superhero and those who are devoted to its demise in their garden.

The garden cure is firmly on the side of the dandelion as superhero, though. Every part of it is edible and the toothed leaves are bursting with vitamins A, B, C and D. In Chinese medicine, the dandelion is seen as something of a cure-all, with the Chinese Pharmacopoeia in 2020 listing 40 patent medicines with the *Taraxacum* genus for use in treating more than 50 diseases. But in the West, it is famous for – and has been since before Culpeper – its diuretic capabilities. The name 'dandelion' comes from the French *dents de lion*, or 'lion's teeth', though no one knows quite why. Its more common name in France is *pissenlit* and in Britain it has always been known, as Culpeper puts it, 'vulgarly', as 'piss-a-beds'.

You have been warned: dandelion is best eaten during the day to avoid the bed situation. The leaves are a very effective diuretic as they increase urine output without depleting potassium levels. The root has been used to support liver function and (also with leaves) for constipation. The roots and leaves contain inulin, a prebiotic fibre that helps beneficial gut bacteria. There is no lack of ways to eat dandelion either. The flowers can be used to make tea or add to a salad, while the leaves (soak overnight to avoid bitterness) are used in salads or cooked as a vegetable (often with bacon). The roots can be grated into salads or roasted to use as a coffee substitute. The dandelion is a multi-tasking plant on every level.

Put on your spectacles for this tale

Eyes, bloodshot

All references to the Doctrine of Signatures should now be filed under 'historical fiction' in bookshops but, in the 16th and 17th centuries, the idea that God created plants to tell us what they could cure was taken very seriously indeed. There were a lot of misses – some of them, such as snakeroot (*Ageratina*), could be fatal – but one that continues to intrigue is eyebright (*Euphrasia officinalis*). It's a small wildflower found growing in grasses and meadows, with white petals that have thin, purple stripes and yellow dots. The flower was thought to look like a jaundiced and bloodshot eye and thus, or so it was said, it would be able to cure one.

'If the herb was but as much used as it is neglected, it would half-spoil the spectacle maker's trade,' wrote Nicholas Culpeper in his *Complete Herbal* in 1653. He advised that taking the juice or distilled water of eyebright in white wine or broth has 'helpeth all infirmities of the eye that cause dimness of sight'. He even noted that it could be a cure for blindness. This is not true, of course, though it was used for centuries to treat minor eye issues such as conjunctivitis. In German, it is called *Augentrost*, or 'comfort of the eyes'.

What to believe then? Eyebright continues to be used by some herbalists, but there is not enough modern evidence to support the idea that it is much more than a pretty wildflower. Some small studies suggest it contains anti-inflammatory and antimicrobial properties that could possibly sooth inflamed eyes, but further and more rigorous studies are still needed. Perhaps the whole tale of this little flower can be summed up by an eye chart:

IT SEEMS THAT
SEEING
IS NOT
BELIEVING
AFTER ALL

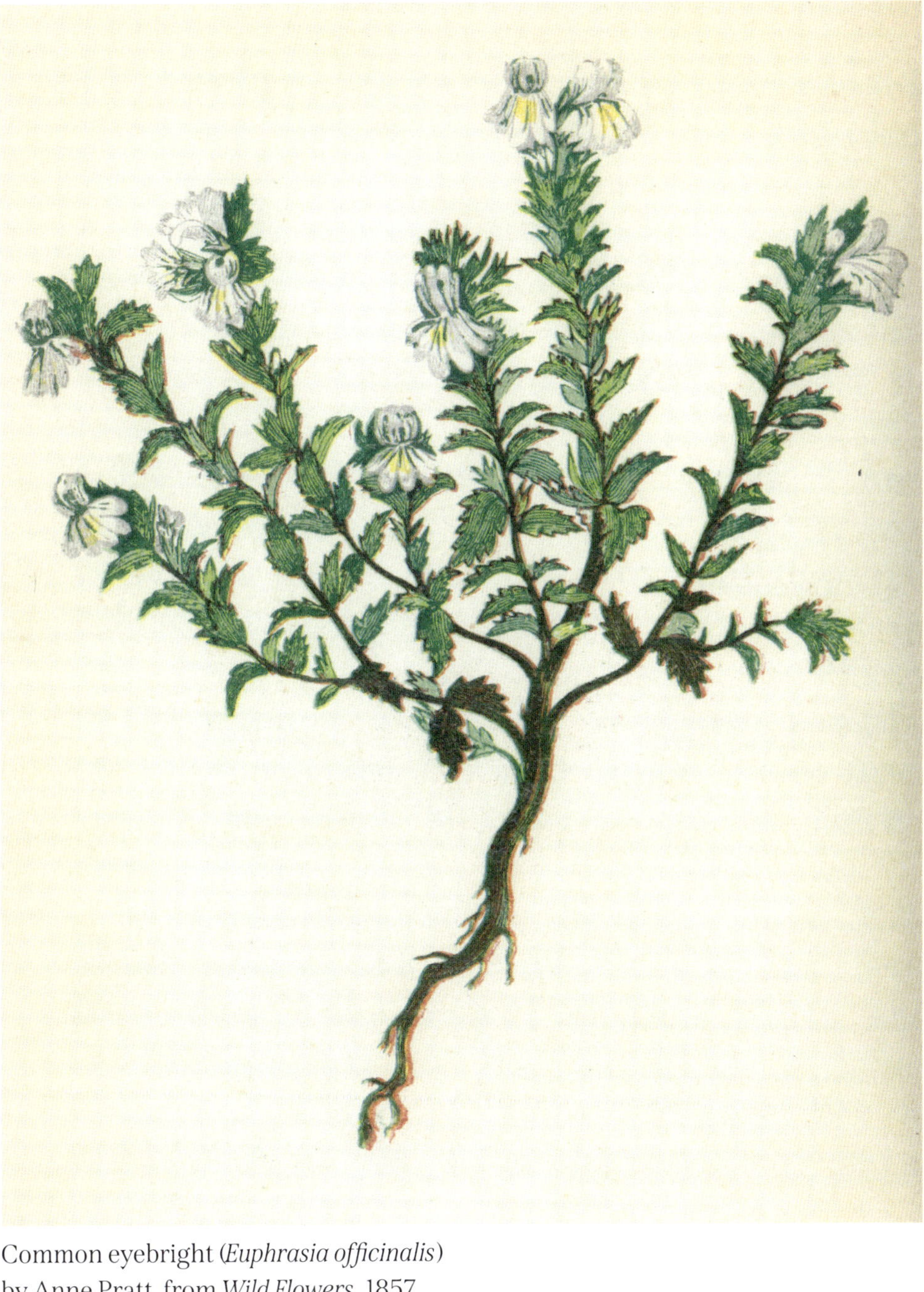

Common eyebright (*Euphrasia officinalis*)
by Anne Pratt, from *Wild Flowers*, 1857.

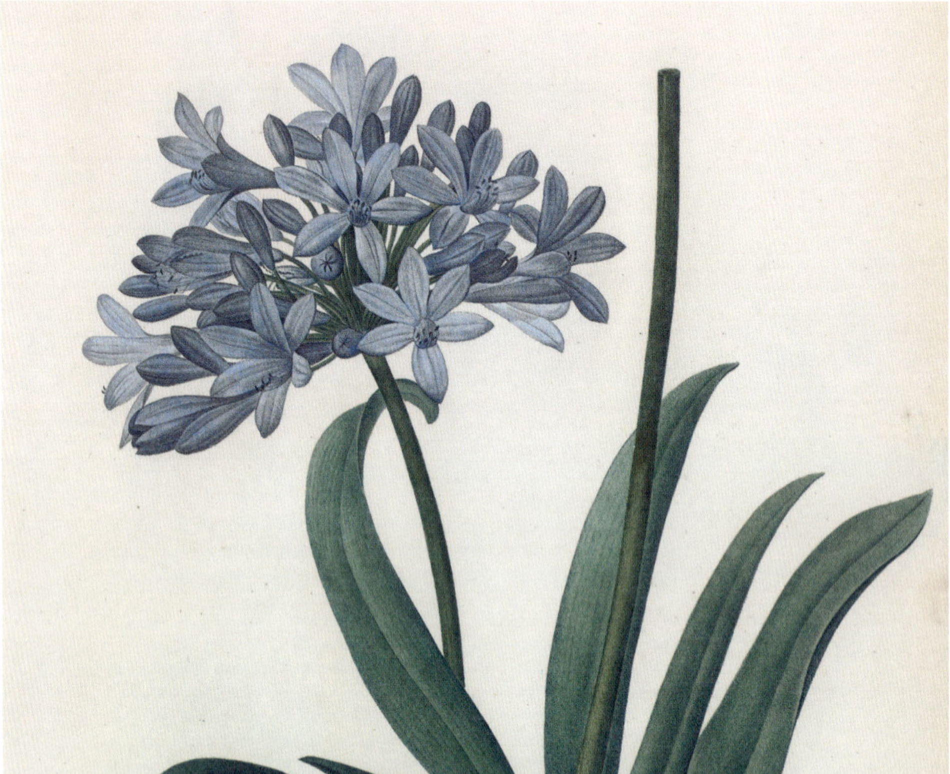

African lily (*Agapanthus*) by Pierre Joseph Redouté, from *Les Liliacées*, Vol. 1, 1802.

There's still a way to have a beautiful garden

Hay fever, treating

It's all about sex really, at least in plant terms. The thing about pollen is that, basically, its job is to travel. It's produced by the male reproductive part of a plant (the anthers at the tips of the stamens) and it needs to go and find – via the wind, water, insects or animals – the stigma or female part of the plant. In some cases, it's a very short trip and in others it's a trek. One US survey reports that wind-borne pollen can travel more than 1,600km (1,000 miles) in 36 hours. But close or far, the point from the plant's perspective is that pollination occurs, which is followed by fertilization and then seeds.

Tom Ogden is an American horticulturist and researcher who became interested in 'allergy-free gardening' because his wife, mother and sisters all suffered from hay fever. He developed his own rating system for which plants are more responsible for allergic symptoms. It's called the Ogden Plant Allergy Scale (OPALS) and, for anyone with hay fever, it's a revelation that allows you to understand which plants are to be avoided and also which plants can make up your garden without resulting in constantly sneezing.

One basic rule: avoid wind-borne pollinators. Because distribution via wind is so random, the male part of the plant, the anther, produces lots of pollen to ensure that at least some of it finds the target. Other plants have simplified things, with flowers that contain both male and female parts, but even then some have less pollen than others. Then there are those that have separate male and female flowers on the same plant, so at least the pollen doesn't have to travel far. Then there are those plants that are dioecious, such as juniper, which have separate male and female plants or, in this case, trees. On the Ogden Scale female junipers score 1 and male junipers are a 10. You know which one to avoid if you have any kind of hay fever at all.

The plants with the lowest pollen are sterile plants and the female version of dioecious plants which have no pollen. But there is also a wide choice of other plants with low pollen ratings. *Agapanthus*, for instance, score 1. Olive trees are a 10. There's a petunia ('Purple Wave') that is a 1. Double hollyhocks are a 2 and singles are a 3. Your goal – if you suffer from hay fever – is to create a beautiful haven for yourself, with the lowest possible score.

The Naked Ladies have been helping for centuries

Gout, suffering from

There is so much to unpack when it comes to the flowers commonly known as 'naked ladies'. They are called this because, in autumn, when you are least expecting them, their largish, lavender-coloured petals pop up overnight. The plants have no leaves, hence the naked bit. They live in 'reverse time', with the leaves coming later. Indeed, it is one of those plants that seems to have created confusion from the start. Other common names are 'autumn crocus', despite the fact it's not a crocus, and 'meadow saffron', despite the fact it has no saffron. The only thing that is clear: naked ladies aren't what they seem.

Linnaeus named them *Colchicum autumnale* after the city of Colchis, which was, in Greek mythology, where the sorceress Medea lived in her garden of magical herbs that included many poisons. Medea herself had her murderess moments, and this is indeed both a cure and a kill plant. All parts are poisonous and it was the weapon of choice used by murderess Catherine Wilson, the last woman to be hanged in England in 1862. She was a nurse whose patients tended to die after they'd changed their wills to include her. She was convicted of only one murder – her landlady Mrs Soames – but is thought to have killed at least six others. Mrs Soames died from colchicum poisoning.

That's the dark side of the story, but naked ladies can also claim to be on the side of the angels. *Colchicum autumnale* has been used since ancient times and was documented in the *Ebers Papyrus* (1550 BCE) as a cure for pain and swelling. It has been packaged in various forms as a cure for gout, and Benjamin Franklin was a fan after sampling Eau Medicinale, a remedy made by French military officer Nicolas Husson in the 1780s. Its corms contain a tricyclic alkaloid, named colchicine, which acts to reduce the inflammation caused by the build-up of uric acid crystals in the joints. It is still prescribed for gout, both to relieve pain and to prevent a reoccurrence, as well as to prevent symptoms of Familial Mediterranean Fever, an inherited inflammatory condition.

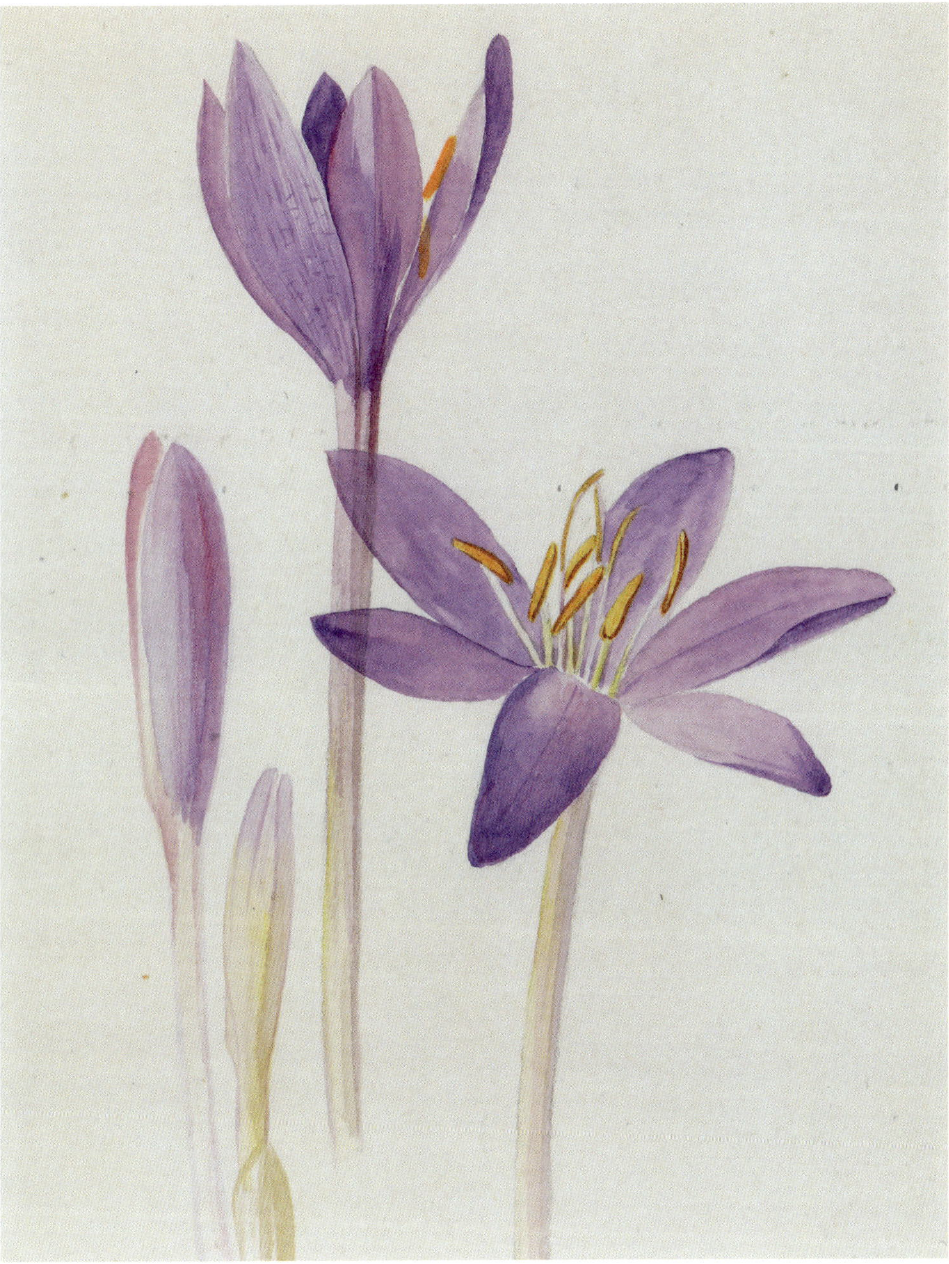

Autumn crocus (*Colchicum autumnale*), watercolour on paper by Lilian Snelling, early 20th century.

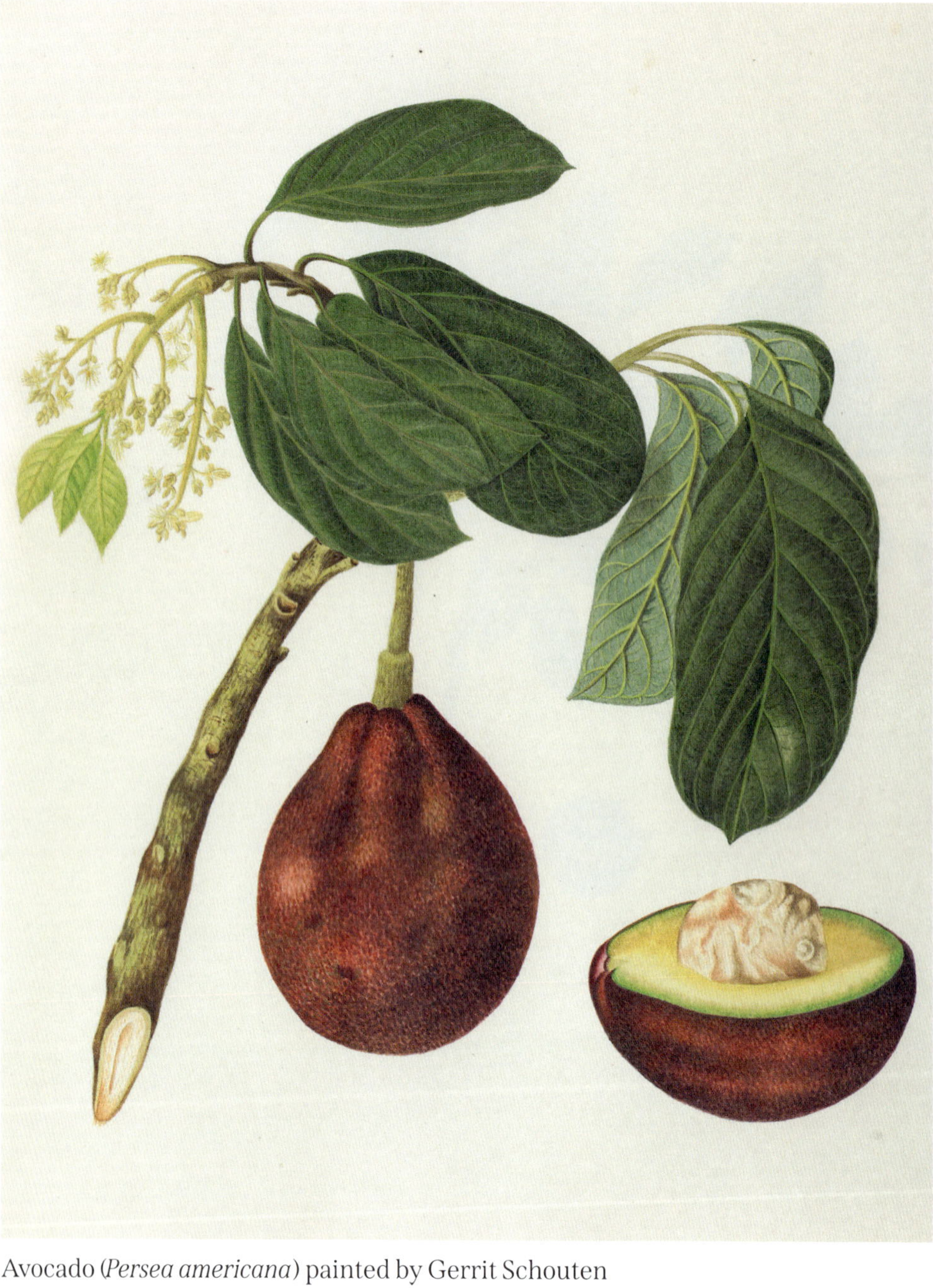

Avocado (*Persea americana*) painted by Gerrit Schouten from the album 'Schouten Surinam Orchids', 1830s.

There's something in plants that can help the good guys

Cholesterol, too much bad

The whole cholesterol drama in our bodies is like an endless Wild West shoot-out. The 'bad' cholesterol (think bandits and robbers) refers to Low-Density Lipoprotein or LDL which, when in excess, leads to fatty plaque build-up in the arteries that can then result in heart disease and strokes. The 'good' cholesterol is High-Density Lipoprotein or HDL (think John Wayne), which then rides to the rescue, helping to remove excessive plaque in your arteries. Bad cholesterol comes from eating foods high in saturated and trans fats such as red meat and fried products. Good cholesterol comes from healthy unsaturated fats such as fish, whole grains and avocados. It's good versus evil, three meals a day, and it's tiring for all concerned.

There's an outside agent, however, which can be called in to help. Think of it as a 'deputy sheriff' type of role. Sterols and stanols (known as phytosterols) in plants are components in cell membranes, providing structure and fluidity. They are constructed in a similar way to cholesterol and, when in the human gut, will compete and ultimately block some cholesterol from entering the blood stream. This means fewer 'bad' guys and a healthier cholesterol balance. Studies show that the overall reduction of baddies is reported to be between 7 and 12.5 per cent.

A large number of plants are required if this is going to be effective. It is estimated that we need 1.5–3g of sterols/stanols a day for this and, though phytosterols are in many types of nuts and seeds, legumes, fruit and veg, it would be almost impossible to achieve this through food alone. For instance, avocados (*Persea americana*) have one of the highest levels of sterols, at 75–100mg per fruit, but that means you would need to eat 15–30 avocados a day. That's a lot of avocados, which is why, instead, people use supplements or buy fortified products, including milk and yoghurts. John Wayne appreciates the support.

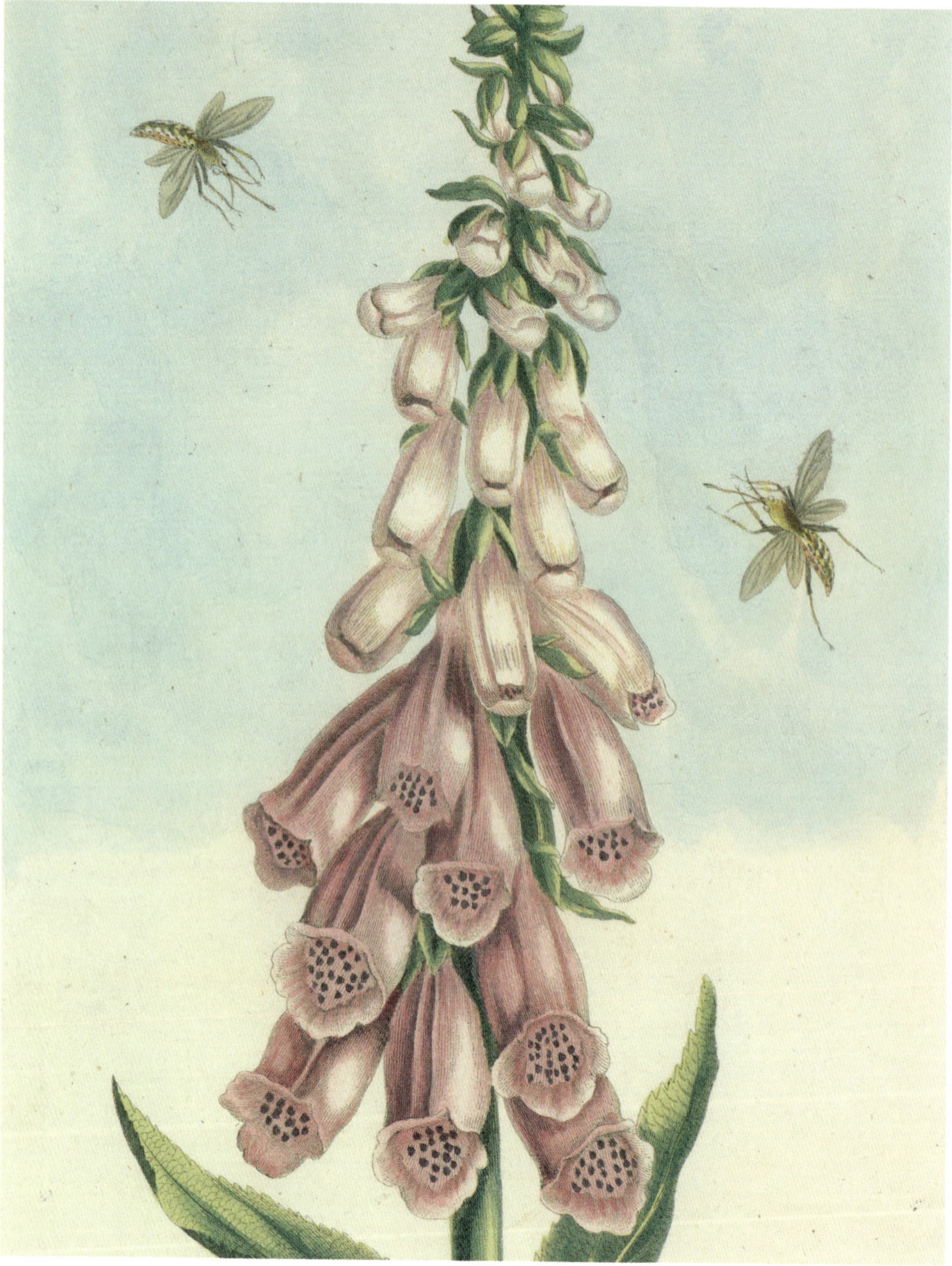

Foxglove (*Digitalis purpurea*) by Pierre Joseph Buchoz, from *Collection Précieuse et Enluminée Des Fleurs...*, Vol. 2, 1776.

There's one man to thank for figuring out the foxglove riddle

Heart failure, treatment for

It used to be known simply as 'the dropsy', which we now call oedema, and is a build-up of fluid in the body that can be caused by congestive heart failure. The foxglove plant had been used for centuries for a variety of ailments, including, as noted by Leonard Fuchs in 1542, as something for the 'scattering of the dropsy'. But its 'discovery' as a cure really belongs to an Englishman named William Withering, a physician and keen botanist who was working in Birmingham in the 1750s, when he was asked by a patient for his opinion on a family recipe for the dropsy:

'I was told that it had long been kept a secret by an old woman in Shropshire, who had sometimes made cures after the more regular practitioners had failed. I was informed also, that the effects produced were violent vomiting and purging; for the diuretic effects seemed to have been overlooked. This medicine was composed of twenty or more different herbs; but it was not very difficult for one conversant in these subjects to perceive, that the active herb could be no other than the Foxglove.'

Withering was a figure who epitomized the English Enlightenment era, a philosophical man with a curious mind and a deep interest in medicine and science. He was a distinguished botanist, the author of a book entitled *The Botanical Arrangement of All the Vegetables Naturally Growing in Great Britain* (1786) and a fellow of the Linnaean Society. This is why he would know, instinctively and logically, that the most important plant in the Shropshire herbalist's concoction had to be foxglove, or *Digitalis purpurea*. He began using it in his practice, embarking on what became a study of foxglove, recording in scrupulous detail its use with 163 of his patients who had the dropsy. His work took the plant from folklore to the realms of science. He found that the dried powdered leaf was the most effective and gave precise details for making an infusion. He also recorded, for the first time, side effects such as nausea and vomiting and the occurrence of green/yellow vision. If these occurred, he said, the dose was to be interrupted and then lowered. He wasn't sure how the drug 'scattered the dropsy' but alluded to a connection between heart failure and dropsy.

Withering published his findings in 1785 as 'An Account of the foxglove and some of its medical uses'. Before this, dropsy was almost always fatal. The paper was received with acclaim, but the use of digitalis continued to be irregular at best, due to fear of the plant's toxicity and the fact it was often used to treat other diseases such as epilepsy (for which it had no effect). Indeed, the painter Vincent Van Gogh is thought to have been treated for epilepsy by his French physician, possibly with digitalis, resulting in 'yellow vision', or xanthopsia, as can been seen in the vivid yellows prominent in his later paintings.

It would be another 100 years before the foxglove's role in treating heart disease would be better understood and for science to reveal that the leaves (*Digitalis lanata* is now used) contain cardiac glycosides which help regulate the heart. *Digitalis*, like many medicinal plants, is both life-saving and a poison, with all parts being toxic (see *Agatha Christie, Too Much*, page 201) and Withering's work was devoted to how to use it for the former. He was a polymath, with many other interests, including chemistry and geology, but in his only known portrait, he holds a foxglove in one hand (not advisable today, of course, due to its toxicity). He deserved to be proud: it was his meticulous work that began a process which changed the treatment of heart disease forever, saving countless lives.

'*Digitalis*, like many medicinal plants, is both life-saving and a poison.'

The cure can be found in a nut that is child's play

Venous insufficiency

The body's arteries and veins are supposed to work as a team: arteries take blood away from the heart, veins bring it back. The relationship doesn't always orchestrate that smoothly, though, and 'chronic venous insufficiency' means, basically, that the valves in your veins are slacking. This can lead to varicose veins, swelling and aching ('heavy') legs. Blood can pool in various places, leading to burst capillaries and skin discolouration.

Riding to the rescue, though the horse in question is a plant and not an animal, is the tree *Aesculus hippocastanum*, aka horse chestnut, from the soapberry family. The tree is native to the Balkans and was introduced to Europe and Britain in the 1500s. Its large, glossy brown seeds (hidden inside spiky, green casings) are used for the children's game of conkers. It's connection to the equine world is not clear, though it is said to have been used in the dim and distant past as a cure for various horse ailments.

A potion with conker shavings was used for centuries as a folk cure for vein problems, and modern analyses and studies have provided strong evidence that horse chestnuts have medical properties that are effective when dealing with the symptoms of venous insufficiency. The nuts contain a saponin known as 'aescin' or 'escin' which, basically, acts to block the enzymes that cause capillaries to leak. The seed extract, applied as a cream, has been shown to soothe varicose veins and reduce inflammation and swelling. A word of warning: the nuts themselves are toxic and are not to be eaten.

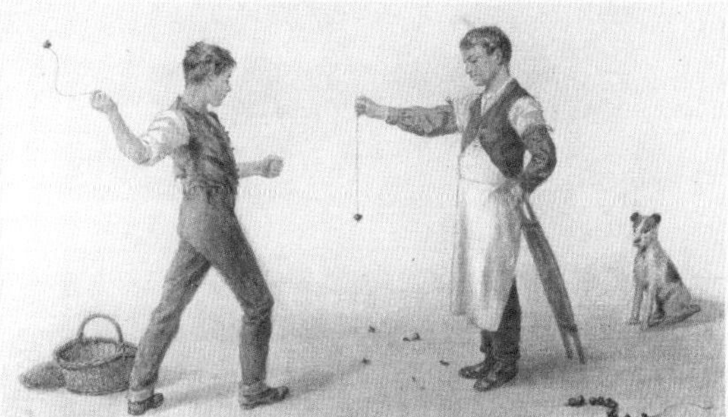

Illustration of boys playing conkers by Henry Robert Robertson, from *Plants We Play With*, c.1900–1915.

The amazing story of the life-saving Madagascar periwinkle

Cancer, treatment of

When you see a periwinkle, you do not think 'cancer treatment superstar'. Instead you might say 'Oh, that's sweet', as it busily goes about its business of filling spaces in the border or container. Its proper name is *Catharanthus roseus*, though it was also known in the past as *Vinca rosea* and, commonly, as Madagascar or rose periwinkle, not to mention old maid and bright eyes. It has evergreen ovate leaves and small, distinctive, five-petalled flowers that (despite its botanical name) can be pink, red or white. In the garden it's a summertime all-rounder: useful for city, courtyard, gravel and cottage gardens, patio and containers, borders and beds, edging, underplanting and ground cover. In other words, it grows everywhere and, though gardeners are grateful for its constancy, normally we wouldn't give it another thought.

The story of the Madagascar periwinkle is a travelogue of almost superhuman proportions. It's native to Madagascar, the fourth largest island in the world, off the eastern coast of southern Africa, but was soon on its way to other places. First, during the golden age of the Swahili trade (8th–15th centuries) it was spread, via cuttings from sailors, around Indian Ocean ports. The first known written record of it dates from 1658 when it was documented in Madagascar by French East India Company governor Étienne de Flacourt who said it was used locally to relieve heart problems and headaches. Before he died, he sent seeds and cuttings to King Louis XV's head gardener at Versailles who, having grown it successfully there, sent some to the head gardener at London's Chelsea Physic Garden.

The perky little periwinkle had already seen empires come and go and, in the 20th century, news about its folk medicinal uses had also spread, probably via the transatlantic slave trade and other means, around the world. A concoction made from its leaves was used in far-flung countries to treat several conditions but mainly diabetes. And it was this that, in the 1940s, attracted the attention of researchers from the University of Western Ontario in Canada and the pharmaceutical company Eli Lilly.

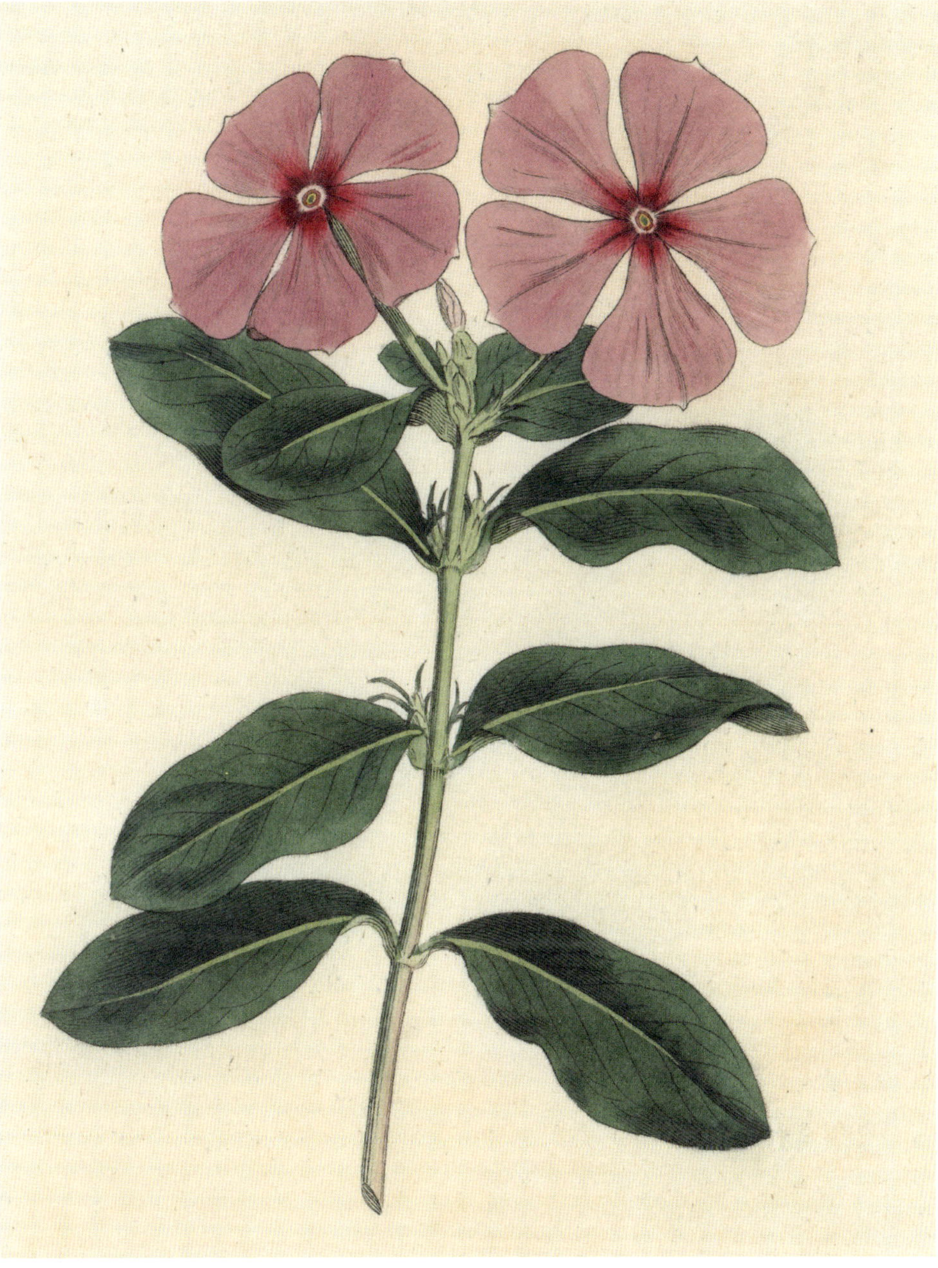

Madagascar periwinkle (*Catharanthus roseus*) by Sydenham Edwards, published in *Curtis's Botanical Magazine*, 1794.

But how did these researchers, in the northern Americas, even know about this folk medicine? This is a question that was also asked by curators at London's Chelsea Physic Garden when researching the history of the plant. The answer, found in a Canadian book on the periwinkle, involves a situation that can only be called a serendipitous masterstroke. It seems that this information can be traced back to a conversation involving Dr Robert Noble of the Ontario team and a Miss Farquharson, who was described as a Jamaican maid or a patient of his brother. She told him how the leaves were used to treat diabetes in Jamaica and suggested they contact a doctor there who duly sent the leaves to Canada.

The two research teams now set to work and found the plant extracts were not very effective in lowering blood sugar levels in mice but that they did dramatically decrease the number of white blood cells. This was the 'Eureka' moment. Some cancers, such as leukaemia, involve a proliferation of white blood cells. It wasn't until 1958 that the plant's key alkaloids, vinblastine and vincristine, were isolated and purified. Both are now cornerstone chemotherapy drugs. Vinblastine stops cell division and is used to treat a wide variety of cancers, including testicular, ovarian, breast, bladder and lung. Vincristine has revolutionized the survival rate of childhood leukaemia.

This is one of those tales – of chance, luck, empire, slavery, folk wisdom and science – that would be unbelievable if it wasn't true. The periwinkle does not give up its secrets lightly and the chemical structures of these alkaloids are still not fully understood. It should come with a warning 'Don't Try This At Home' because, in the raw, all parts are toxic, but research continues into its life-saving mysteries. In the meantime, in its day job, this unassuming little flower continues to perk up gardens around the world. But the next time you see that small blast of pink, give the periwinkle a nod. It has saved countless lives.

‘This is one of those tales – of chance, luck, empire, slavery, folk wisdom and science – that would be unbelievable if it wasn’t true.’

A powerful treatment that exists due to serendipity – and graft

Ovarian and breast cancer, cure for

This is a story of heroic endeavour and determination, and it all began on a hot August day in 1962 when a botanist named Arthur Barclay spotted a 7.6-m (25-ft) Pacific yew in a small stand of conifers in the Gifford Pinchot National Forest in the American state of Washington. He was working for a branch of the US Agricultural Research Service on a needle-in-a-haystack joint operation with the National Cancer Institute, which involved taking random samples from plants that would then be screened for anti-cancer properties. The tree was given a designation of B-1645 (it was the 1,645th sample collected by Barclay) with samples taken of stem, fruit and bark.

The yew tree has an ancient and rich history, mostly to do with death and war. It is poisonous and its wood was used to make weapons by the Egyptians, the Greeks and Romans. The star yew in almost any story is *Taxus baccata* or English yew. In yew terms, the Pacific species, *T. brevifolia*, was always seen as an also-ran: it lived in the shadow of the conifer giants of the Pacific Northwest, growing very slowly, attracting no attention. Loggers considered it a 'weed' tree, compared to the in-demand Douglas fir, and so it carried on, unnoticed and (it must be said) unloved.

The bark sample, in the laboratory, showed anti-cancer activity. This is why, in September 1964, Barclay returned to visit B-1645 to collect 14kg (30lb) more bark. Most laboratories weren't interested in taking on the project as, in most instances, similar plants that have the capacity to kill living cells just kill everything, cancerous or not. But one man, Monroe Wall, the chief scientist at the Research Triangle Institute, was undaunted as he and colleague Mansukh Wani had previous experience of a cytotoxic plant that yielded promising results. In 1966, he and fellow researchers managed to isolate a compound from the yew bark and named it Taxol, but attempts to find its characteristics proved difficult. It became a 'low priority' project but, eventually, Wall and Wani discerned its molecular structure and published the results in 1971.

In a movie, this would lead to a breakthrough but, in real life, what followed was an impasse. The yew bark was difficult to obtain and there

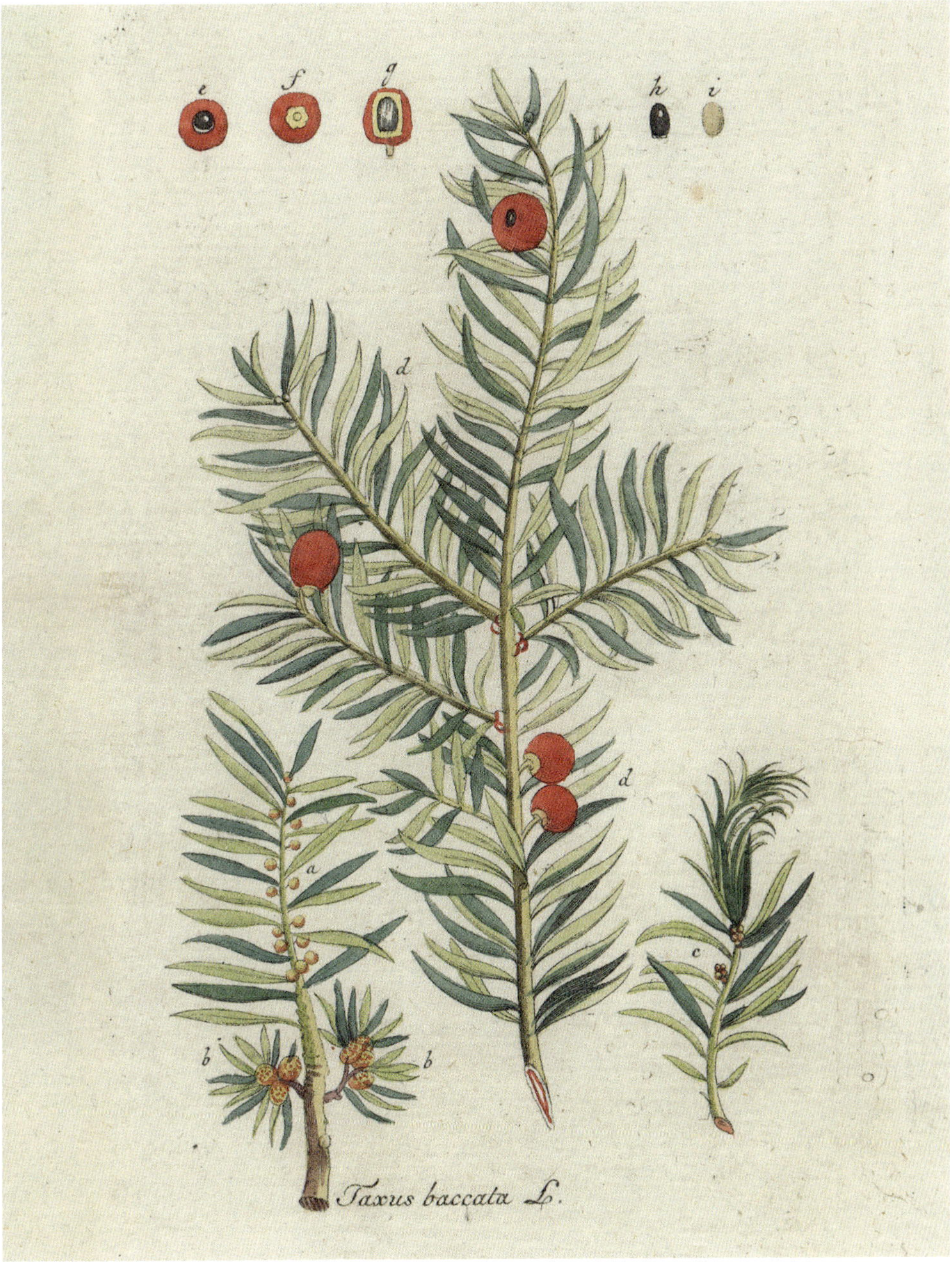

English yew (*Taxus baccata*) by Johannes Zorn, from *Icones plantarum medicinalium*, Vol. 6, 1796.

was also the fact that, without bark, the tree would die. At the time, it took six trees to provide enough bark to obtain half a gram of Taxol. In 1978, however, research showed that Taxol had the ability to regress mammary tumours in trials with mice, and interest was revived. Susan Horwitz, a molecular pharmacologist at the Albert Einstein College of Medicine in New York, took on the task of finding out how Taxol actually worked.

Horwitz's first hurdle was to get more Taxol. She'd only managed to obtain a few milligrams and in 1979 she wrote to the National Cancer Institute to ask for more Taxol. This was achieved but at a cost: 3,200kg (7,000lb) of bark were collected, killing 1,500 trees. Environmentalists were outraged, especially as the trees were part of the Pacific Northwest's old growth ecosystem forests and they feared that worse was yet to come. The stage was set for a 'Conservation versus Cancer Cure' battle.

Back in New York, Horwitz had discovered that Taxol worked via a mechanism new to researchers. Most anti-cancer compounds work by inhibiting cell division. Taxol worked in the opposite way: it caused the cells to turbo-charge themselves and, in the process, they became unable to co-ordinate cell division. In the end, this caused cell death. Her results were published in 1979 and, once again, hopes were raised that a miracle drug had been found.

The initial problem with human trials, though, was how Taxol could be administered. It wasn't soluble in water. Cue more research which found that Taxol would dissolve in a potion involving a derivation of castor oil and ethanol known as Cremophor EL. Clinical trials were able to begin in 1983, but there was an immediate crisis when one of the first patients died of anaphylactic shock. For five years, trials were suspended as scientists worked out how to avoid allergic reactions to Cremophor EL. New protocols were devised involving patients being pretreated with steroids and giving the drug over a 24-hour period. In 1988, human trials restarted.

Results were more than promising, especially with ovarian cancer. It wasn't until now that the issue of the trees was faced. Even for treating ovarian cancer patients, hundreds of thousands of Pacific yews would have to be felled – and demand would only increase in the future. How to get Taxol, though, without the bark of the Pacific yew? Scientists scrambled themselves once again. First it was discovered that the needles of *Taxus baccata,* or English yew, yielded a similar compound to Taxol, but it would still need a synthetic addition. All in all, it took years, and more science, but a semi-synthetic procedure for producing Taxol was devised.

Finally, all the pieces were in place. Only one practical obstacle remained. The National Cancer Institute is a US government agency and, to make the drug marketable, it needed a drug company to come on board. The deal was done with Bristol-Myers-Squibb. In December 1992, Taxol was approved by the US Food and Drug Administration, first for ovarian cancer and later for breast cancer and non-small cell lung cancers.

It had been 30 years since botanist Arthur Barclay had stood in the middle of a forest in the Pacific Northwest and decided to remove some bark from a Pacific yew. His 1,645th specimen turned out to be that one golden needle in the haystack. It took three decades for us to understand nature's complicated chemistry and to find a way to administer it to people. This story, recounted in various aspects by cancer and scientific bodies, has so many twists, turns and leaps, and multiple times when failure seemed the most likely outcome, but the appliance of science saved the day. Taxol is now used around the world and, since 1992, it has saved hundreds of thousands of lives and will continue to do so, forevermore.

'This is a story of heroic endeavour and determination.'

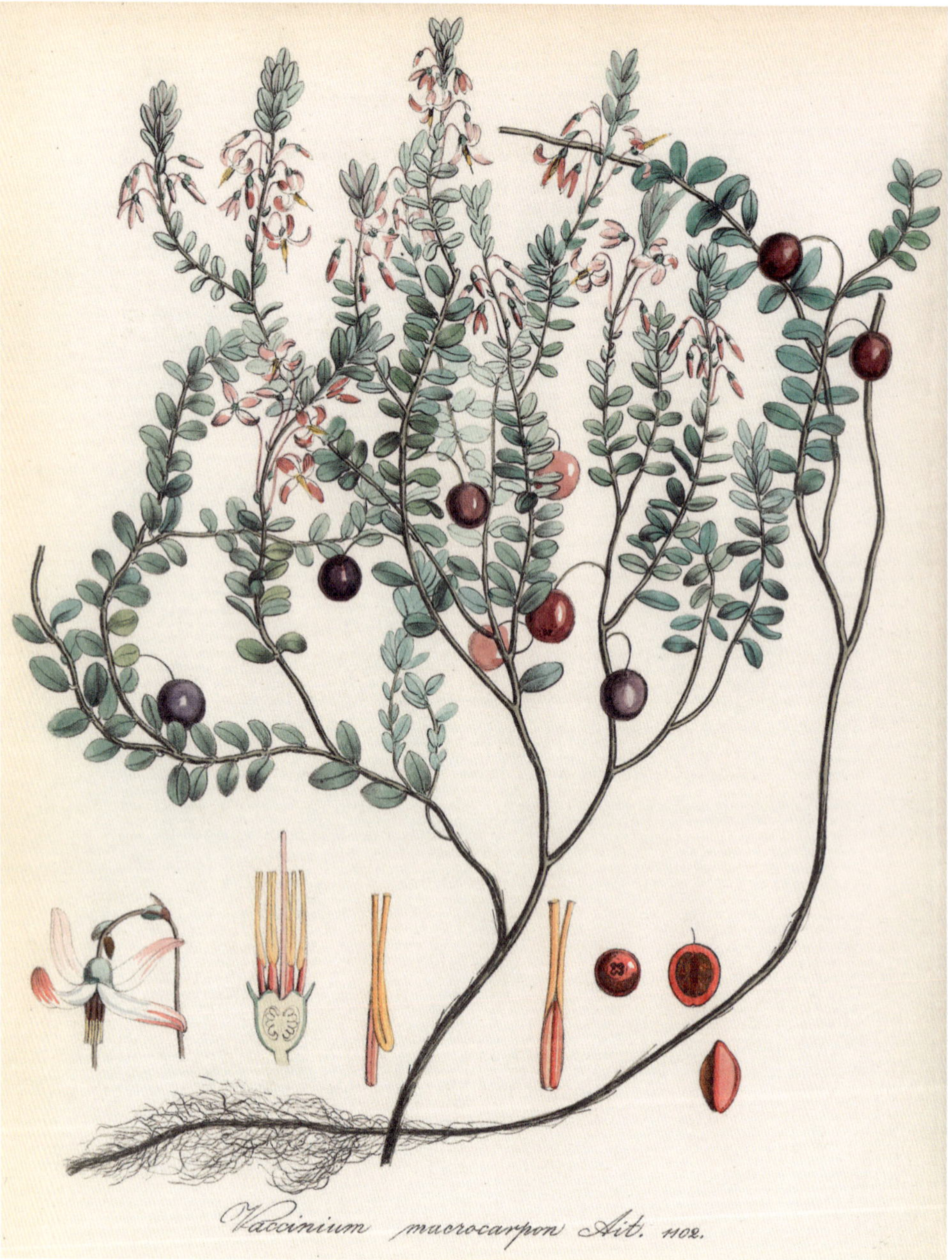

Vaccinium macrocarpon by A. J. Kouwels, from *Flora Batava*, Vol. 14, 1872.

There is one plant that can stop it taking hold

Urinary tract infection

Cranberries are considered a superfood but that is not their superpower. The plant (*Vaccinium macrocarpon*), native to North America and used extensively by Native Americans in food and medicines, produces berries that are high enough in antioxidants that they out-rank the likes of broccoli or spinach. They are also rich in vitamins A, C and K, as well as flavonoids, which are the good guys in reducing chronic disease risks. The downside? They are tart to the point of sour and, when picked, are quite hard. The plants love acidic and very moist (as in boggy) soil. Native Americans used to pound cranberries with lean meat from bison or elk and mix with tallow to make pemmican, a precursor to the high-energy snack bar.

None of these, though, touches on their superpower which hinges on the fact that they contain a high concentration of A-type proanthocyanidins, or PACs. Other plants such as grapes and other berries contain B-types. The A-type has been shown to block *Escherichia coli*, the bacteria that commonly causes urinary tract infections, from being able to attach itself to the lining of the bladder. Cranberries are now accepted as a way to prevent cystitis from taking hold and have also been shown to decrease the number of symptomatic urinary tract infections over time. As it happens, in the garden they are also quite handy, providing year-round interest with pink spring flowers, green foliage that turns yellow and red in autumn, and bright red berries in winter.

There's one plant with a particularly sleepy reputation

Insomnia, dealing with

There is no definitive description for insomnia and how it differs from minor sleep problems. Symptoms include both not being able to fall asleep, and waking up and not getting back to sleep during the night. The closest to a description could be someone who has trouble sleeping at least three nights a week over a period of three months. Insomnia is thought to affect between 10 per cent and one in three people. That's a lot of people up in the night, feeling anxious about it. The sleep industry is in perpetual overdrive to produce a variety of sleep potions and lotions, pills and machines.

Many plants have reputations as sleep aids. Lavender (*Lavandula*), St John's wort (*Hypericum perforatum*), red Korean ginseng (*Panax ginseng*), chamomile and kava-kava (*Piper methysticum*), to name a few. One of the most persistently prevalent is common valerian (*Valeriana officinalis*), which has tall stems and white flowerheads with many tiny blooms loved by bees. It is known as a herb with calming and sedative properties and has been studied many times for its effectiveness in treating insomnia and/or anxiety. The results of the studies seem to be conclusively inconclusive, as they are difficult to compare, involving different concentrations and settings. However, that has not stopped the European Medicines Agency approving valerian as a traditional herb to aid sleep, and valerian dry ethanol extract being recognized as a herbal remedy for improving sleep.

It is not fully understood how, or why, valerian works. Researchers are still evaluating its compounds and the mechanism involved. It is known that GABA (gamma-aminobutyric acid) is a major inhibitory neurotransmitter (think of it as an 'off switch') in the central nervous system. Its receptor GABA-A is the key player for many drugs that aim to help sleep (these include benzodiazepines such as Xanax and Valium). Valerenic acid and valerenol, compounds found in the root, have been shown to bind to GABA-A receptors and could be behind its sleepy reputation. Three things of note: valerian has been around as a sleep aid for centuries and certainly since ancient Greece; it smells pungent and has been described as 'stinky socks'; and cats love it, as, like catnip, it makes them have too much fun.

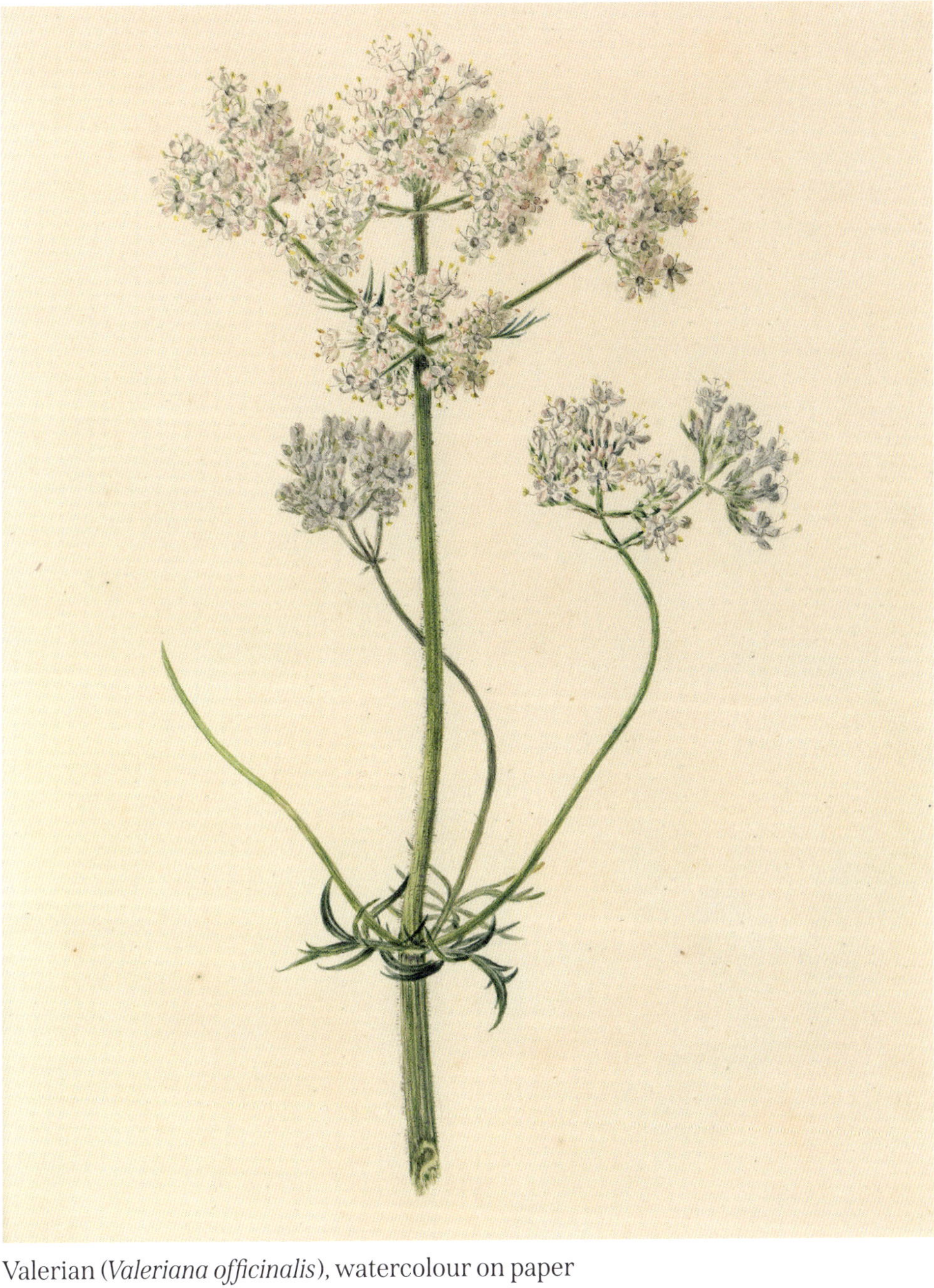

Valerian (*Valeriana officinalis*), watercolour on paper (artist unknown) from *Flore du Desert*, Vol. 2, *c*.1800.

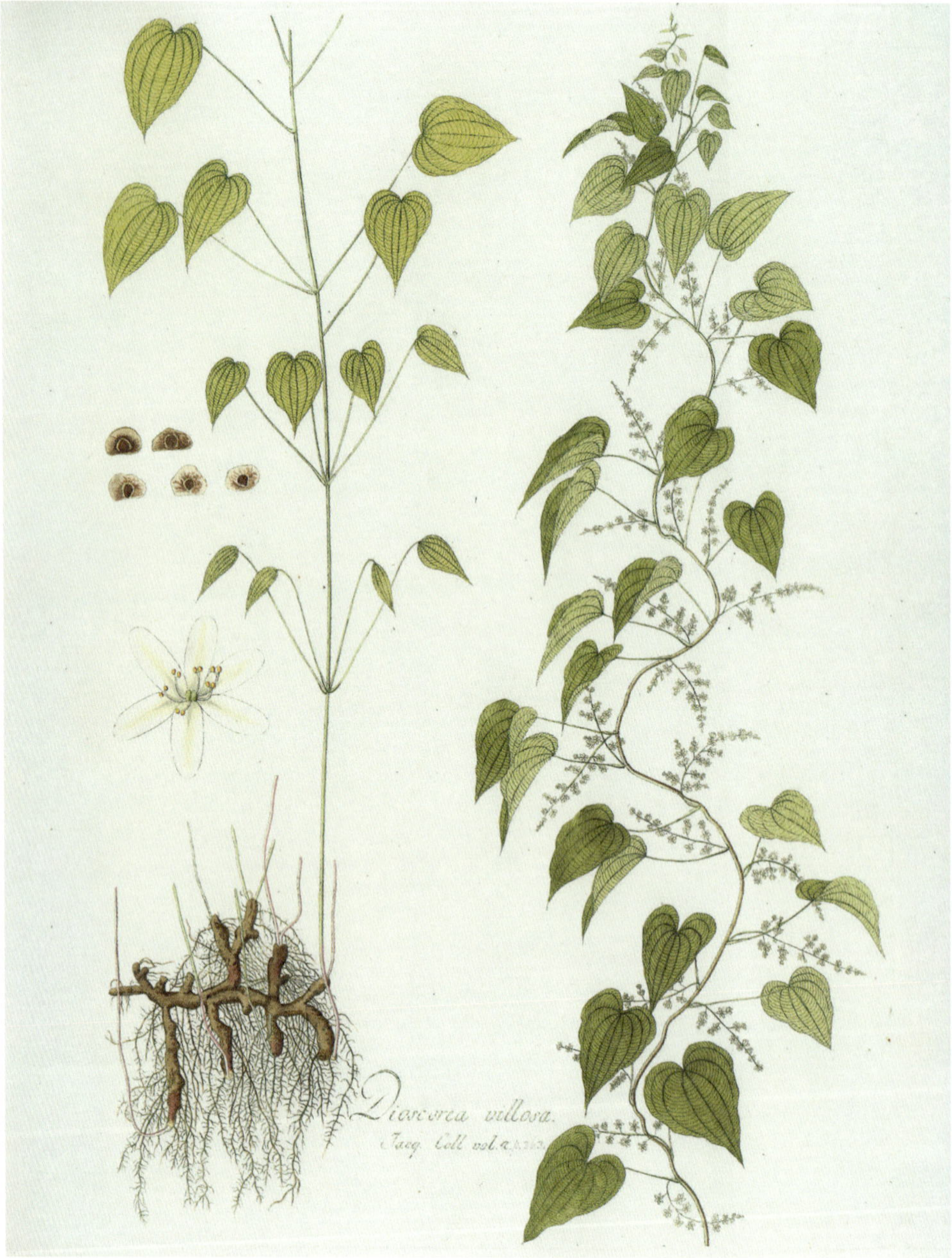

Wild yam (*Dioscorea villosa*) by Nicolaus Joseph Jacquin, from *Icones plantarum rariorum*, Vol. 3, 1781–95.

Who knew that the humble yam could be so helpful?

Menopause, navigating

It used to be that only a brave few women discussed the menopause in public. Now it can feel as if everyone is talking about it. This is a very good thing for a subject that felt almost taboo, leaving women to struggle on, feeling alone, with the likes of profuse night sweats, brain fog, severe mood swings and depression. The menopause occurs in women when the female hormones oestrogen and progesterone start to decrease, signalling the end of reproductive life. Some women have only mild symptoms, but others are affected severely. For many, hormone replacement therapy or HRT is life-changing. In the past, HRT was a crude construct, consisting of synthetic hormones and a mix of equine oestrogens from pregnant mare urine. It now involves body-identical hormones made from plant sources, mainly soya bean and yam plants, which are then converted in a lab to have the same molecular structure as the female hormones.

The humble wild yam (*Dioscorea villosa*) and soya bean (*Glycine max*) contain phytohormones with similar molecular structures to human hormones. The roots of the wild yam, a twining vine with heart-shaped leaves, contain diosgenin, which is essential for synthesizing hormones, while the soya bean has certain isoflavones that are rich in phytoestrogens. The key word here is 'synthesizing'. The chemical compounds are transformed in the lab into body-identical hormones. Self-prescribing by eating tonnes of soya beans and wild yams is not going to work. (By the way, this wild yam is not classed as edible anyway as it can cause nausea.)

There is no lack of herbal remedies out there for the menopause. Black cohosh (*Actaea racemosa*), red clover (*Trifolium pratense*) and hops (*Humulus lupulus*) are some of the many plants packaged up for menopausal symptoms. Black cohosh, also known as bugbane due to its insect-repelling smell, is a North American native that is thought to help with hot flushes, though the mechanism for this is not understood yet. Red clover has many isoflavones, which may also reduce hot flushes. There is no miracle cure here to report, although there have been multiple studies into these remedies, with dozens conducted for black cohosh alone, but results remain decidedly mixed.

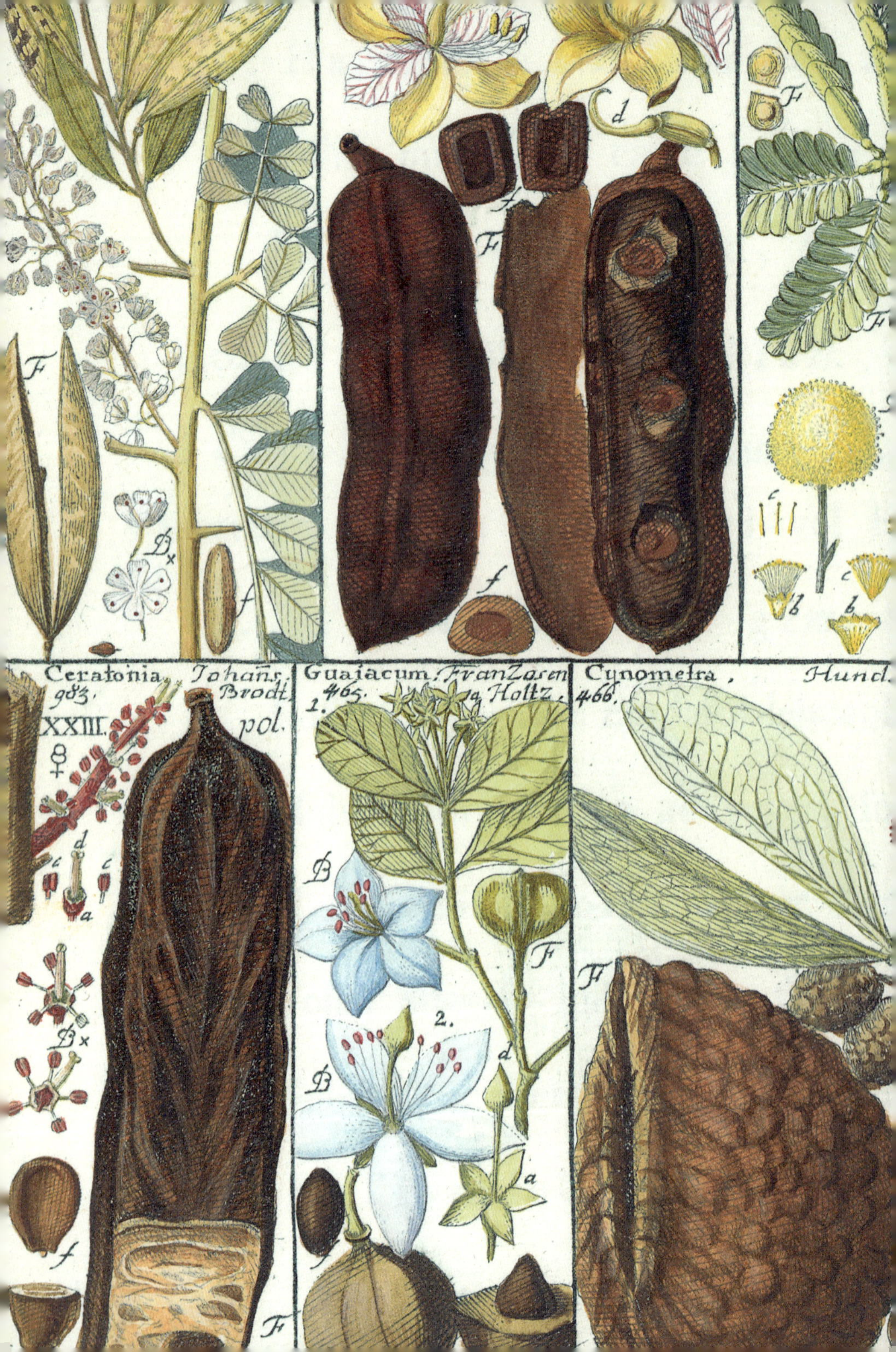
Ceratonia
983.
XXIII.
Johans.
Brodt
pol.
Guaiacum.
465.
Franzosen
Holtz.
Cynometra.
466.
Hund.

Chapter 2

MIND

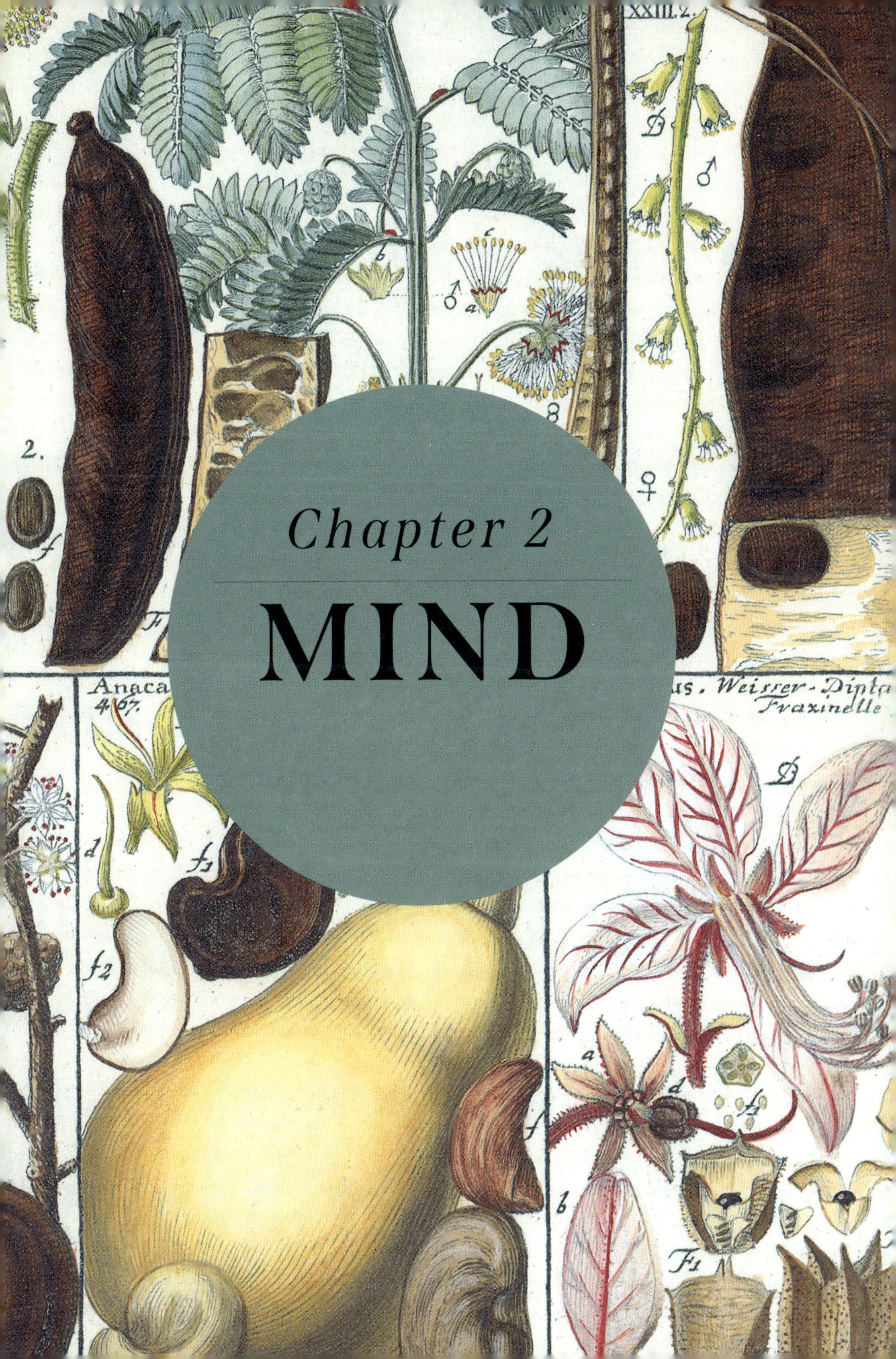

The cycle of life is there to be cultivated

Death, fear of

It is easy to assume that most of us are afraid of our own death, even though, as Benjamin Franklin noted, the only things said to be certain in this world are death – and taxes. The fear of taxes is another thing entirely (see *Taxes, Fear of*, page 175), but here we are dealing with death. Studies vary, but they show that between 20 per cent and 50 per cent of us fear our death, though very few suffer from the extreme version of this, thanatophobia, which involves carrying an intense anxiety about it.

What studies do not show is how many people who are gardeners fear their own death. This is an oversight, but it would make sense for the percentage to drop dramatically. This is because the cure for a fear of death is to be a gardener – to see, up close and personal, down in the dirt and up on the ladder, the facts of life as illuminated by a garden. For this purpose, we are going to repurpose Ben Franklin's quote, which he won't mind because he was an avid gardener himself. Here's the gardener's version: 'The only thing that is certain in a garden is death – and sex.' There is also beauty, of course, at least in most gardens, but that is by the bye.

The cycle of life is there for all to see in the garden: seeds germinate, plants grow and mature, wither and die. There is even a rather sonorous word for the process of dying: senescence. A few trees, especially some clonal ones, defy the odds and try to live forever, but they are very much the exceptional exception. The plant that perhaps personifies the cycle of life the most is the corn poppy (*Papaver rhoeas*): it self-seeds at will, thriving in both garden beds and patio cracks, in fields of wildflowers or rubble, as well as those that have been war-torn. Its papery petals are a vibrant red, its centre a bristle of black. In senescence it creates a globular seedhead, with a tiny crown on it with even tinier openings for seeds to escape. One poppy dies and scatters seeds, so that many more can live, flower and die. They are a powerful symbol of remembrance for those who have died in war. In our gardens, they remind us of the cycle of life and how each phase can be seen as equally beautiful.

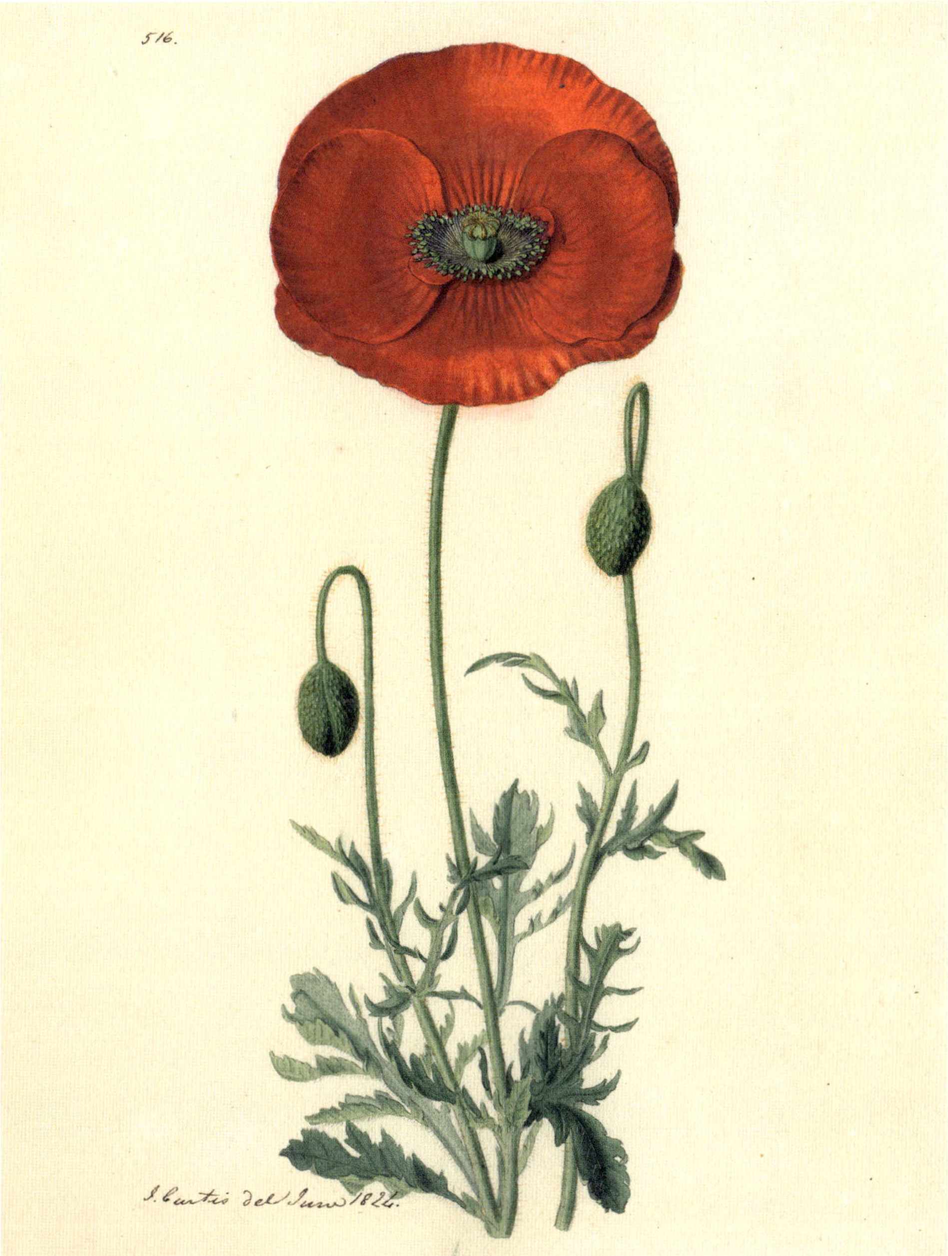

Corn poppy (*Papaver rhoeas*), watercolour
on paper by John Curtis, 1824.

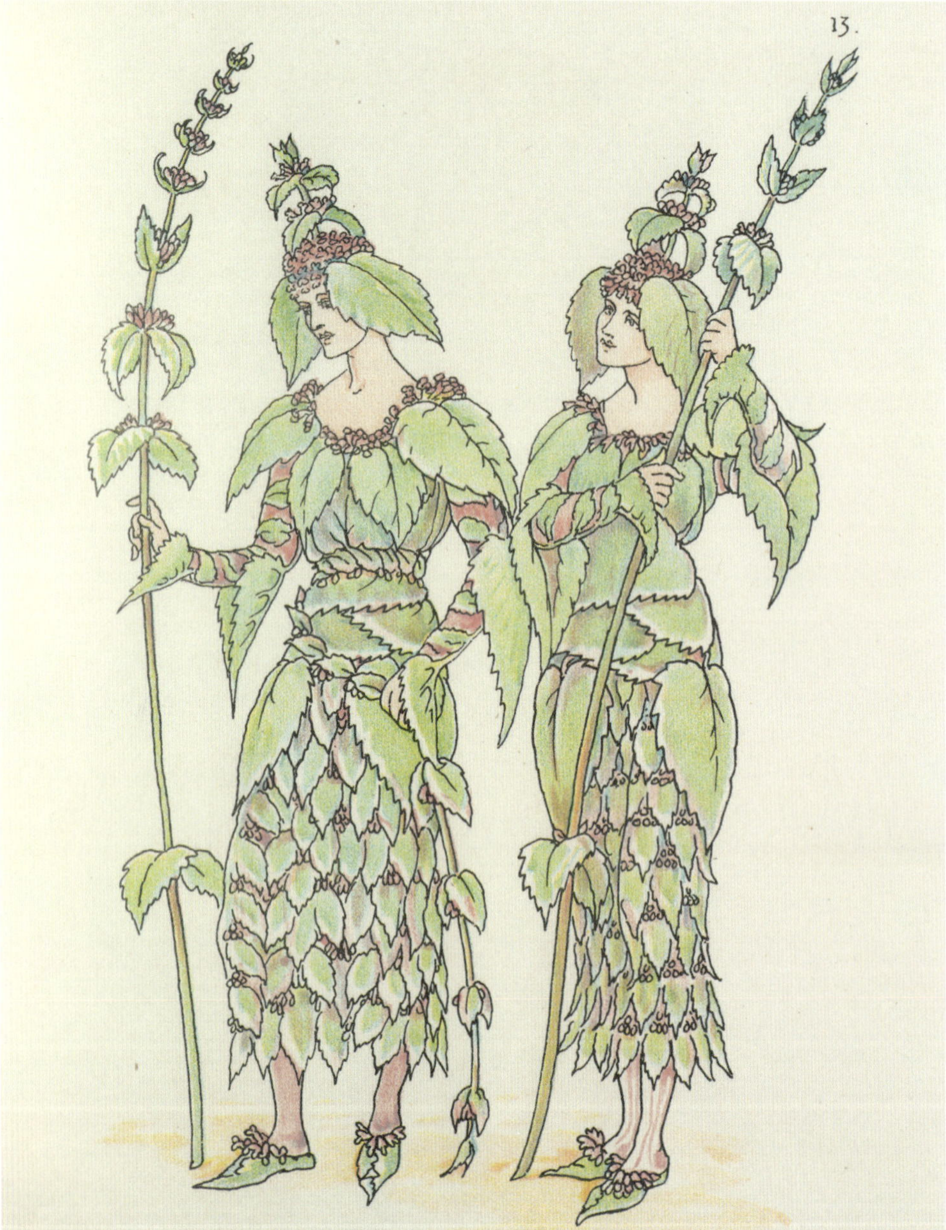

Mint (*Mentha*) by Walter Crane, illustrating *The Winter's Tale* in *Flowers from Shakespeare's Garden*, 1906.

You'll find the antidote in minted condition

Mice, fear or dislike of

Most of us know that if the cat is away, the mice will play, but the question here is: where, exactly, are they playing? Most of us expect a mouse or two (there is never just one) in the garden, but when they decide to come inside and join us at home, that is something else entirely. If you have a dislike or fear of rodents, even cute cartoon ones, then it's important to find their weak spot and in this case it is right in front of our noses. That is because it *is* their noses or, to be more precise, their olfactory receptors. Mice have an acute sense of smell and they also have a secondary organ for detecting smells: the vomeronasal pathway. All of this explains why mice, unlike humans, depend more on their sense of smell than vision.

Forget cheese (at least for now). The garden cure for mice is mint. The stronger the scent, the better, so use the good old-fashioned peppermint (*Mentha × piperata*) or spearmint (*Mentha spicata*). We love mint for many reasons. It makes a soothing tea and a wonderful jelly. There's mint cake, wafers, sweets of all shapes and sizes. It's a one-plant assault on bad breath, which can't be a bad thing. The key to all of this is menthol and that is why it is the enemy of mice. That mentholated aroma – clean and green, some would say bracing – can overwhelm the cold receptors in those tiny mice nasal passages. Think brain freeze but in a nose. It is disorientating and they react by avoiding it.

The battle begins with cotton wool balls soaked in peppermint oil. Place these in spots (inside) where you think you've spotted a mouse: in the eaves, attic or skirting boards. When mopping the floors, add a drop of peppermint oil to the washing liquid, just to let them know you know they're around. You can also bring in pots of the stuff, if you want it. In the garden, especially around tulip planting time, plant up pots of mint and place them in a 'ring of menthol' around your bulbs.

How to remember the one you love, if not where your glasses are

Forgetfulness, tackling

The little blue flower known as forget-me-not, or *Myosotis sylvatica*, self-seeds with romantic abandon in gardens, creating hazy clouds floating just above the ground. It makes for a wonderful 'underskirt' to the likes of tulips and has been a symbol of love since the Middle Ages. In Old French, it was called *ne m'oubliez mye*, and in Middle High German, *vergiz min niht*. As legend has it, a German knight was gathering flowers on a river bank for his true love when he lost his footing and fell into the water. As he was swept away, he threw his bouquet, crying 'Forget me not!' In general, gardens are places where you forget things (such as what time it is, for instance), but let's turn this little blue flower into a particularly pretty mnemonic device. If you want to remember something or someone, visualize it (or them) falling into a river, throwing forget-me-nots back at you. Alternatively, you could write it down – but where's the fun in that?

'In general, gardens are places where you forget things (such as what time it is, for instance)...'

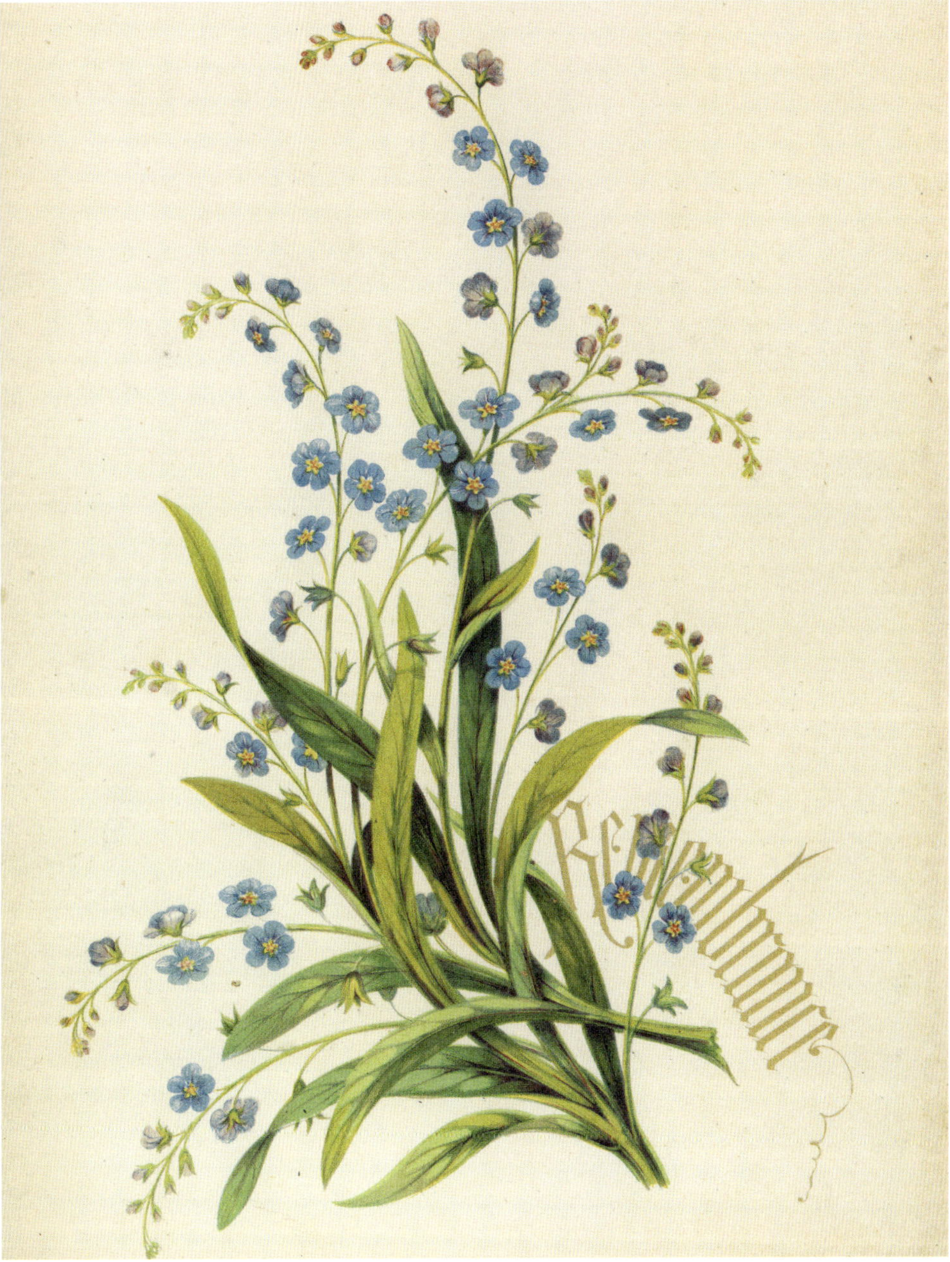

Forget-me-not (*Myosotis sylvatica*) by Owen Jones, from Mary Ann Bacon's *Flowers and Their Kindred Thoughts*, 1848.

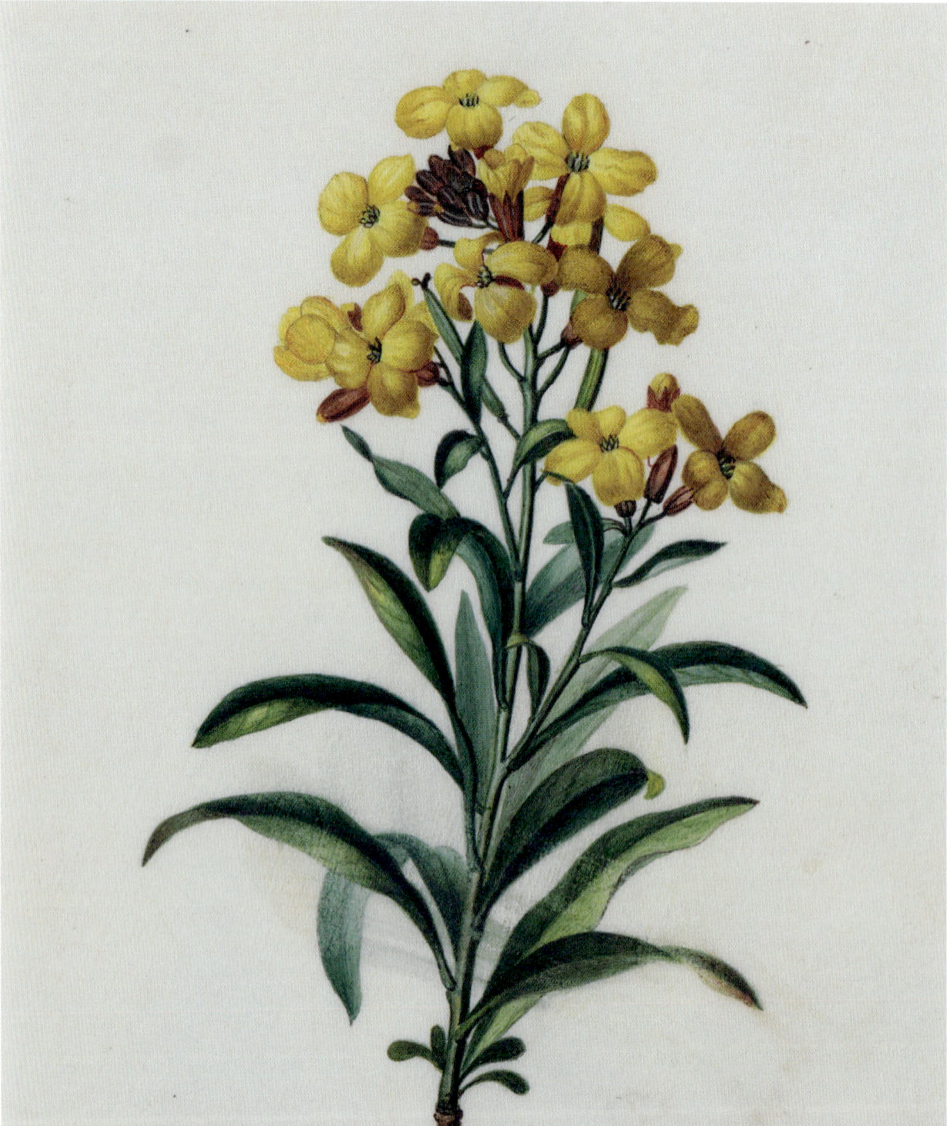

Wallflower (*Erysimum cheiri*), watercolour
on vellum by Pierre J. F. Turpin, *c*.1800.

There is much to learn from the original wallflower

Shyness, prone to

The wallflower is native to southern Europe, particularly the Mediterranean region, but it has never let a little thing like geography stand in its way. It now lives happily, or so it always seems, with its cheerful little flowers, on most continents. This is a rock-and-roll plant in every way, as it loves any sort of stony wall or crack. It is likely that it came to England via the Normans and the story goes – and it's one that keeps on being told and can't be checked – that its seeds arrived in England with the Caen limestone that William the Conqueror imported to build his castles from 1066 onwards.

Wherever it goes – and clearly it goes where it wants – *Erysimum cheiri* is a plant that makes itself useful in many ways. Its delicate scent could hide the unpleasant smells of medieval life and, medicinally, it was seen as a cure for just about anything (heart, sore throat, liver, impotence, menstruation, constipation, pain and fever, and so on). It was one of the first flowers painted in London's Chelsea Physic Garden by illustrator Elizabeth Blackwell in 1737 (see *Married, To A Scoundrel*, pages 191–2). By the time it was realized the wallflower wasn't a cure for just about anything, it had escaped into the gardens – and hearts – of people both rich and poor.

You will find wallflowers now in gardens galore, front and back, as well in some famous ones such as Monet's celebrated Giverny. There, they are elevated to painterly heights, used by the master Impressionist in shades of orange, pinks, bronzes and golds on the west side to emphasize the effects of the setting sun. They are useful and valued, as well, for their long flowering period, scent and for attracting butterflies and hummingbirds.

All gardeners should plant some wallflowers but especially those who are told they are too shy. The next time anyone calls you a wallflower, tell them it is an honour. Then go where you want, do what you want, and be loved by all.

Here's a small cure that has big results

Stress, need to reduce

It's stressful even to think about how stressful life can be and this, immediately, brings us to the subject of cortisol. This is the 'stress hormone' and it's essential to helping us cope in a crisis, regulating blood pressure, controlling our immune system and facilitating sleeping well. We all have cortisol and a healthy pattern would see it peak about 30 minutes after we wake up and then decrease throughout the day until hitting bottom while sleeping. But daily life is full of crises, small and large, and the resulting prolonged cortisol spikes disrupt this daily pattern, which has all sorts of unhealthy consequences.

This is why the stress hormone itself is becoming such a source of stress for us and why all sorts of cures – from mindfulness to meditation to hula-hooping lessons – are deployed in the name of stress reduction. Here's something a lot simpler, though, which came out of a two-year study conducted by the Universities of Sheffield, Westminster and Virginia (in the US), plus the RHS in Salford in Greater Manchester.

People were given some plants for their (bare) front gardens and then the researchers measured what happened next. They were given two large containers and a tree, a shrub and a climber, as well as an assortment of flowering plants and bulbs. These included the likes of some rather old-fashioned favourites such as azaleas, clematis, lavender, daffodil bulbs and petunias.

Cortisol patterns were measured before and after the plants arrived. They showed that, after the new gardens were in place, those with a healthy pattern increased from 24 per cent to 53 per cent. Plus the new gardeners reported a significant decrease in how they perceived their own stress levels and said they felt happier, more relaxed and closer to nature. They also said that just seeing the plants, and flowers, made them feel more cheerful.

This garden cure is a perfect example of 'petunia power'. You may see it as a minor intervention, with a small number of plants, but it's had a big impact on how people feel. Petunias may be small, but they can pack a punch.

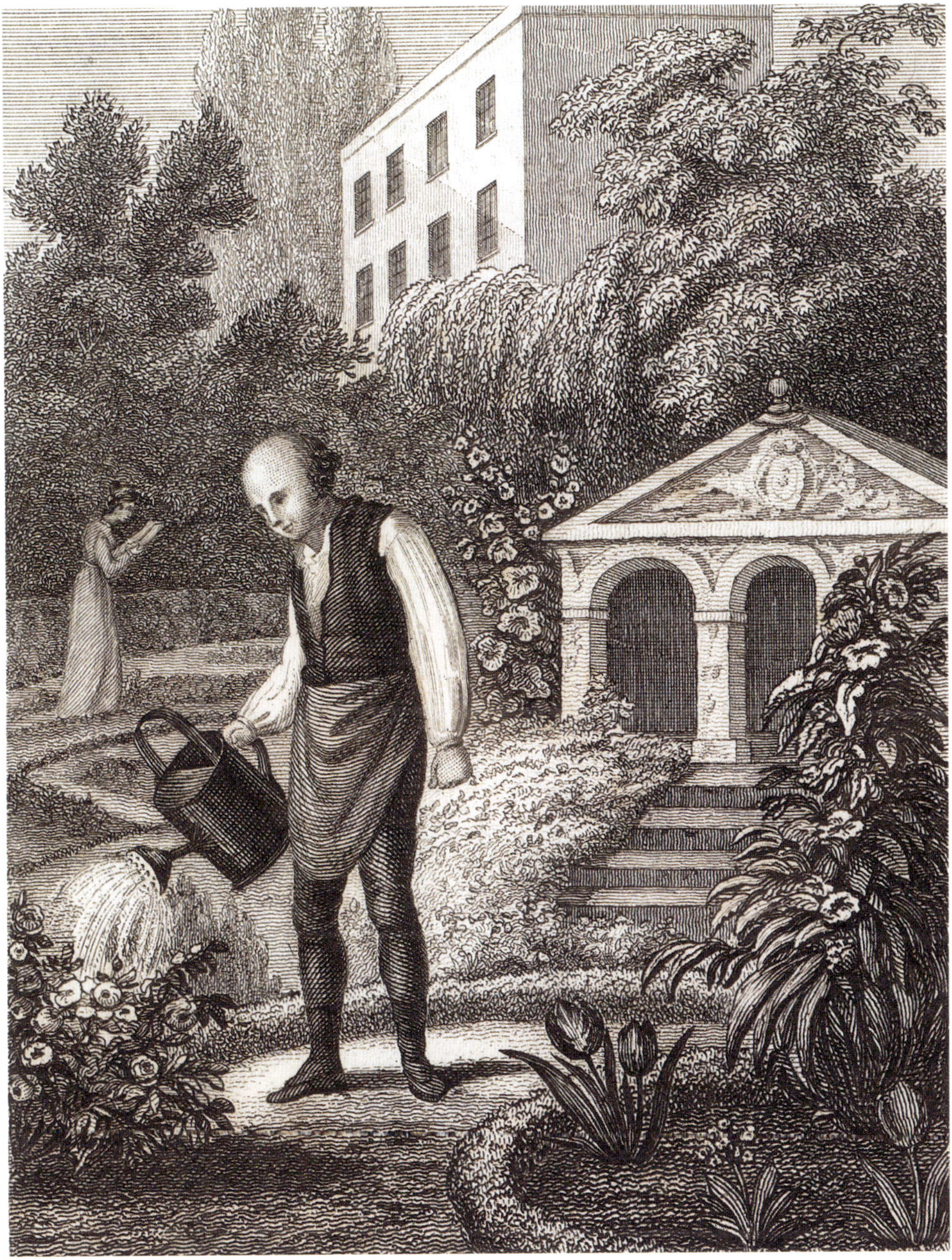

Frontispiece, drawn and engraved by John Shury, from Thomas Mawes' *Every Man His Own Gardener*, 1859.

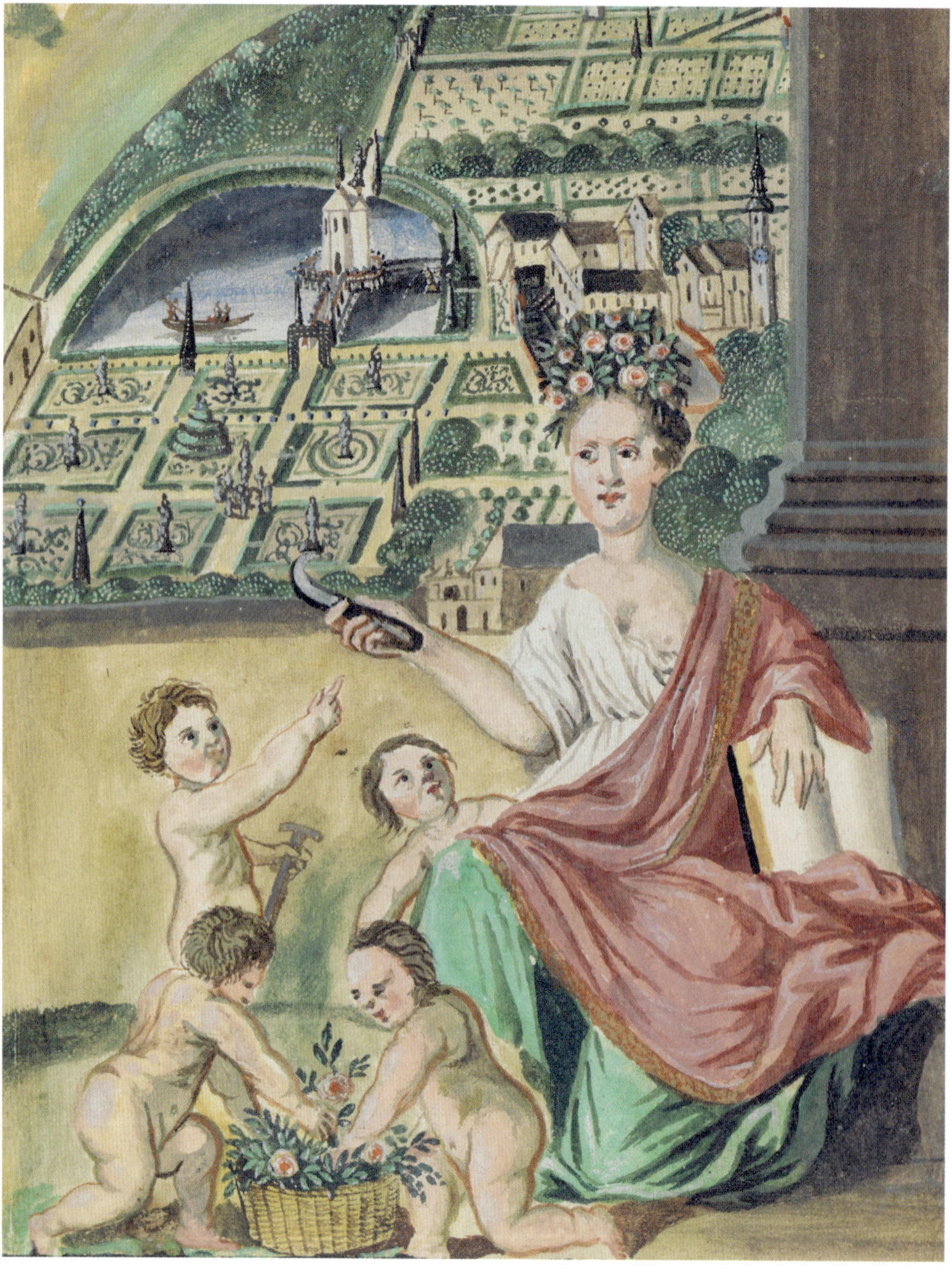

Illustrated title page by Frans George Beissner, from the *Stephenson Clarke Albums: Dutch Garden Flowers*, Vol. 2, *c*.1680.

You are not alone if you want to garden clothes-free

Naked, desire to be

Not all nudity has to happen on a beach, you know. At least that's what seemed to be the motivation of Mark Storey, a consulting editor of the now defunct magazine *Nude & Natural*, and friend Jacob Gabriel, when they came up with the idea of World Naked Gardening Day (WNGD) in 2005. It's always on the first Saturday in May, except in New Zealand when, presumably for weather reasons, it's the last in October.

As one headline said: 'Pants Down, Rakes Up'. It's not an overly organized event, but Storey, who lives in Seattle in the American Northwest, has done the occasional interview. He's a fan of nudity in general. 'It's hard to describe, but anybody who's gone skinny-dipping knows how pleasant it feels,' he told *The Seattle Times* in an article that was accompanied by a photo of him mowing the lawn in the nude (a strategic leaf blocking our view). He says his wife also likes gardening clothes-free. Crucially, their garden is well fenced. 'I don't think a whole lot of people are checking us out.'

Apparently, gardening is second to swimming on the list of family-friendly activities people are most willing to consider in the nude. 'Gardening has a timeless quality, and anyone can do it: young and old, singles or groups, the fit and infirm, urban and rural. An elderly lady in a Manhattan apartment can plant new annuals in her window box,' explained the WNGD website. 'Families can rake leaves in their backyard. Free-hikers can pull invasive weeds along their favourite stretch of trail. More daring groups can make rapid clothes-free sorties into public parks to do community-friendly stealth cleanups.'

It's all supposed to be fun, though not all law enforcement officers would see it that way. Privacy is key and hedging is obviously helpful. Another danger is interminable jokes about 'trimming bushes' and 'weed whackers'. There's also no lack of advice on using shears (keep them above the waist) and to make sure you avoid thorns. As Storey says: 'You don't cut blackberries when you're buck naked.'

There's one aphrodisiac with a reputation that won't go away

Frisky, desire to be

Chocolate, but not as we know it, has had a sexy reputation for thousands of years. It comes from the pods of the cacao tree (*Theobroma cacao*), which is a rather fussy grower, even in its native South America, and, until only a few hundred years ago, it was something that you drank. The original drink was called *xocolatl*, developed by the Mayans and Aztecs, which means 'bitter water'. It was made by crushing the beans into a powder, then mixing it with water and chilli peppers. It was 'frothed' by passing it from one cup to another. Chocolate was revered by the Mayans (they were buried with it) and the Aztecs (where it was reserved for male soldiers and the elite to drink during rituals and before battle). Most famously, the Aztec emperor Montezuma II drank it before having sex with his wives and many mistresses. He is said to have drunk 50 cups a day, each from a new golden goblet. It's hard to imagine he also had time to run an empire.

The first European thought to have drunk xocolatl was the conquistador Hernán Cortés at the court of Montezuma II from (as to be expected) a golden cup. It made its way back to Spain and, along with it, its reputation as an aphrodisiac. The drink, sometimes now sweetened with cane sugar or honey, became popular among the elite as well as the frankly libertine and salacious. Casanova was a fan, as was the Marquis de Sade. Royalty employed their own personal chocolatiers. The first 'chocolate house' opened in London in 1657, with others such as White's following suit – these establishments soon became a magnet for appallingly behaved aristos.

All of this and chocolate still hadn't been made into a solid bar form yet. That happened in 1847 when Joseph Fry produced the first moulded chocolate bar in Bristol. Milk was first added in the 1870s by a Swiss chocolatier. Gradually, over the centuries, chocolate and its reputation have been both refined and democratized. The drink that was seen as magical and only for the elite and the warrior (and forbidden for women by the Aztecs) has become something that is now universally consumed as well as seen as connected to romance and, by default, sex. There are many

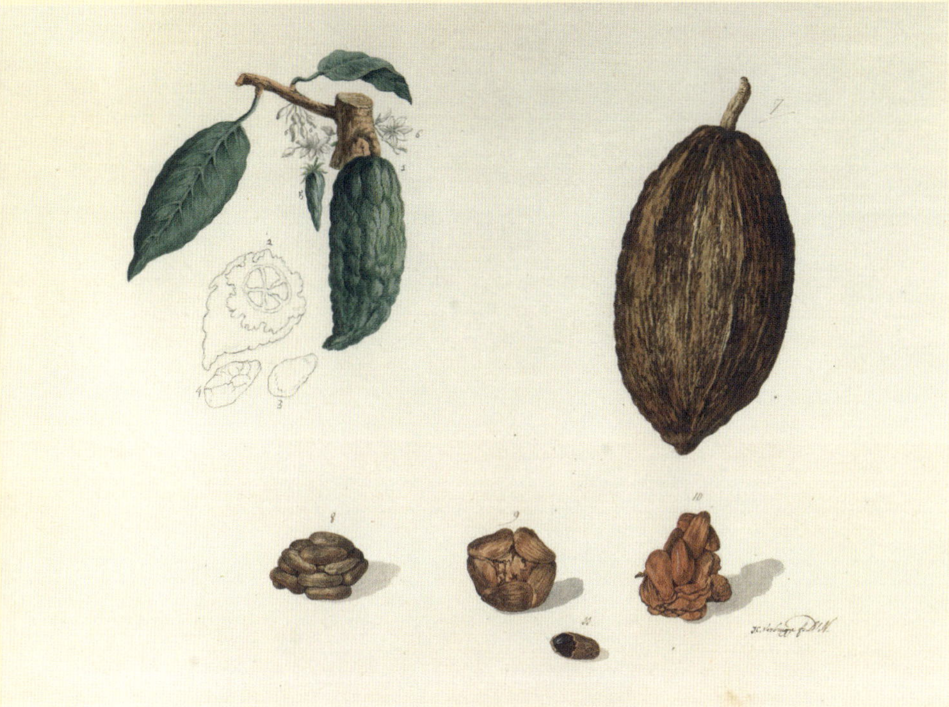

Cocoa bean (*Theobroma cacao*) by Jean Charles Verbrugge, from *Règne Végétal*, Vol. 2, *c*.1800.

plants that enjoy a reputation for putting us 'in the mood' – figs, saffron, ginseng, strawberries, and so on – but chocolate is the most enduring (not to say profitable).

Multiple studies have been undertaken to see if chocolate can induce friskiness, as Montezuma II claimed, though none has been conclusive. What is known is that it does contain phenylethylamine, a monoamine which has been called the 'love molecule' because it is released by the brain during that euphoric period when people are falling in love. However, the amount in chocolate is too low to put anyone in the mood. Then there's tryptophan, an amino acid which is involved in producing serotonin. These two together could be a promising combo, but studies cannot confirm this. Will chocolate make us feel frisky? It has a reputation going back thousands of years and that's got to be worth something. Right?

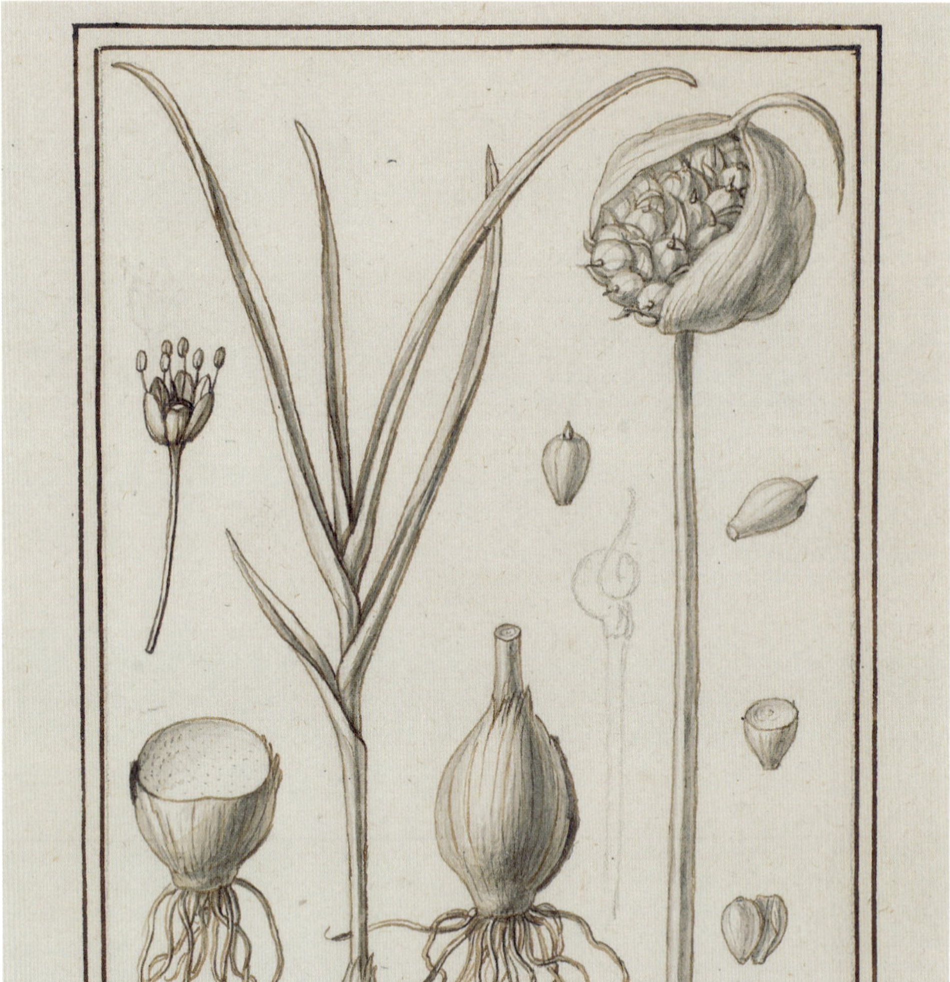

Garlic (*Allium sativum*), pen and ink on paper by Claude Aubriet, *c*.1700.

You suffer from a fear of vampires

Sanguivoriphobia, fighting against

Vampires, aka The Undead, are humanoid creatures who need to drink human blood to stay 'alive'. They often have fangs (all the better to bite) and are nocturnal, as sunlight weakens them. They may indeed be mythical, most probably based on folklore from the likes of the Balkans in the 1700s, but they have been very much kept alive by Hollywood and writers such as Bram Stoker. His Count Dracula may be the most famous, but there are plenty of others, including Spike (à la Buffy), Lestat de Lioncourt (Anne Rice novels) and, of course, Vampire Grandpa Simpson of cartoon fame.

Vampires are so bad they are good (at least for the box office) but not, of course, if you suffer from sanguivoriphobia. Ways to fight them include putting a stake through their heart and decapitation. You can also carry a large mirror or crucifix. But a far less frightening, and ultimately much more portable, anti-vampire remedy can be found in the garden.

Plant garlic! Lots of it. Vampires have an acute sensitivity to strong odours and all garlic (*Allium sativum*) has exactly that. It's also quite versatile, used as a flavouring and for medicinal properties. It contains the chemical compound allicin which is an antibiotic. Another plus is that it is also an excellent pest repellent that will keep mosquitoes away.

The two main types of garlic are hard neck and soft neck (a very sensitive area for all things vampiric). The hard neck has larger cloves with a stronger flavour but doesn't store well. The soft neck has smaller cloves and a milder flavour but a longer storage life. It would make sense to grow both: hard neck first and, when that fades, fall back on the store of soft neck.

More good news for vampire haters: garlic is easy to grow and needs minimal maintenance. You start with cloves, not seeds, and plant outdoors in the autumn as it likes a cold spell to form a good bulb. It can also be grown in pots, but you may want more than one container. Think of this as a very inexpensive vampire burglar alarm. Can you ever really have enough?

The garden knows all too well what it feels like to be under attack

Enemies, too many

Do you often feel surrounded by enemies? Are there people at work who think they can do your job better? Does your family constantly correct? Do you sometimes suspect that your partner is not entirely on your side? And what about that friend who talks behind your back? Does your child disrespect you, your car refuse to start, your dog reject your commands?

That feeling of being surrounded by foes is something that the garden knows all too well. Who'd be a plant? Enemies include wind and rain, freezing temperatures, snow, sun and drought. The soil may be too rich, poor, acidic, alkaline. They may be planted in the wrong location: why, a fern may wonder, did anyone think I would like a sunny corner? Then there are other stresses such as having to share space with a gnome or being dug up by a squirrel.

Thankfully, the garden can also provide a cure. Think laterally. That is what is required when a plant, such as broad beans, must fight back against hordes of blackfly, which are as relentless an enemy as there is. Sometimes the best way to attack is to not attack at all but to distract and divert. This is why there is something called the 'sacrificial crop', which, in the case of blackfly, is nasturtiums. This cheerful, self-seeding annual, *Tropaeolum majus*, originally from Chile and Argentina, is handy on several fronts: it's easy to grow, has pretty flowers that are edible (peppery) and seedheads that can be used as a poor man's caper. But its most important aspect, in terms of our battle, is that it attracts blackfly. Nasturtiums take on the blackfly, so the beans don't have to. (Other examples of companion planting include protecting tomatoes via basil or marigolds, or planting carrots near leeks or onions to confuse carrot fly.) The next time you are surrounded by enemies, ask what you can do (or who you can ask) to distract them. Dangle something attractive in front of them and, if they take the bait, they will soon forget about you.

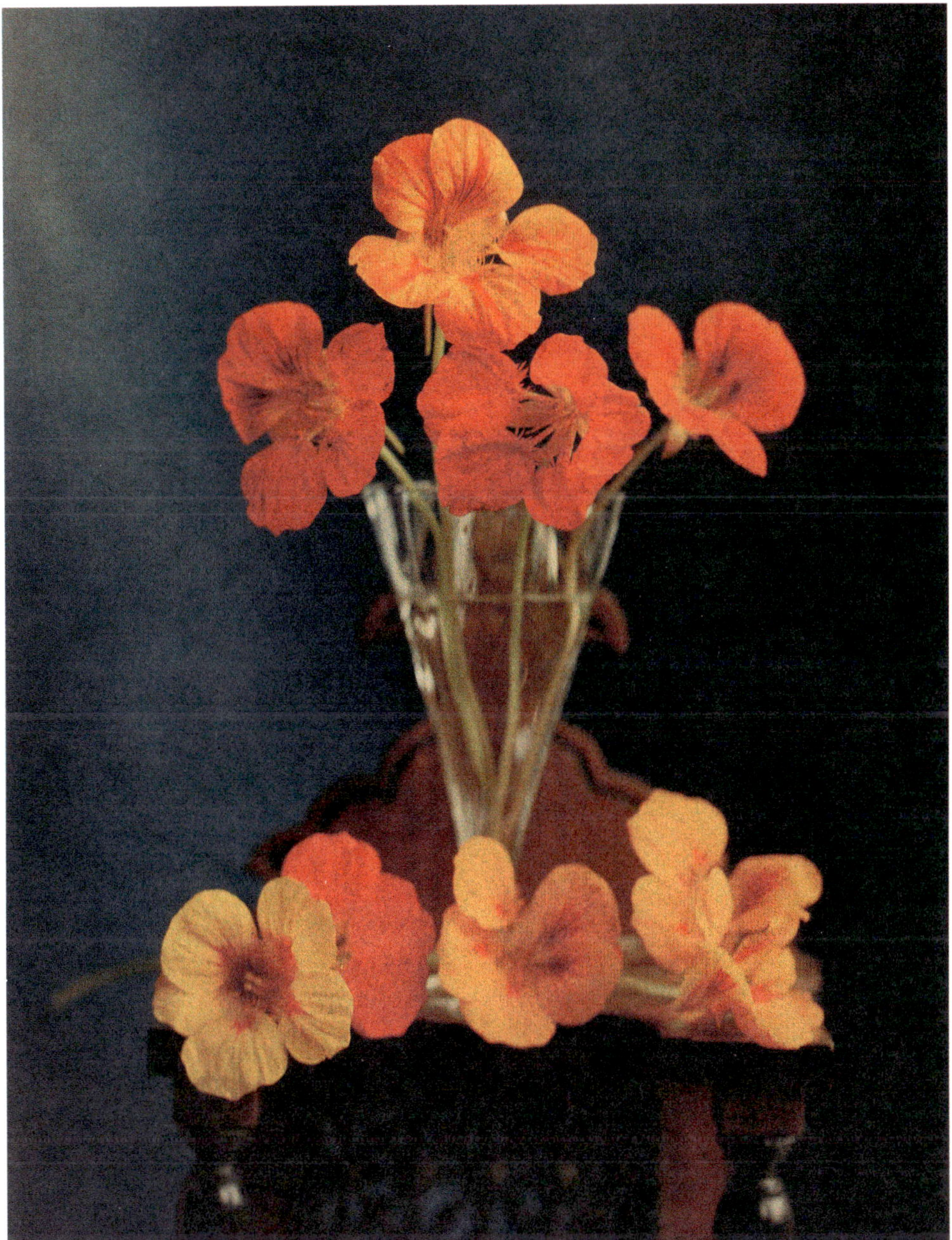

Nasturtium (*Tropaeolum majus*)
by William Van Sommer, 1913.

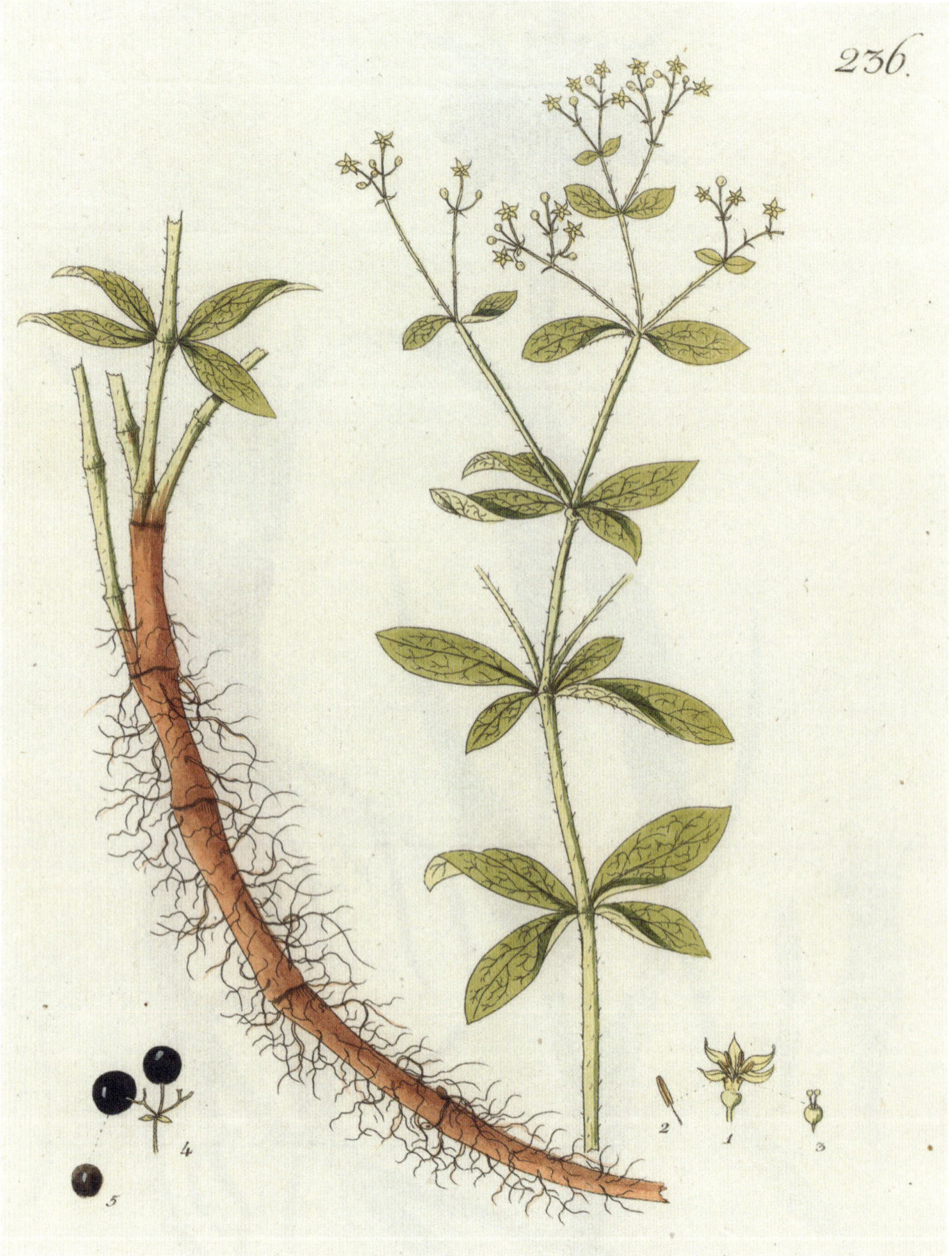

Madder (*Rubia tinctorum*) by Johann Simon Kerner, from *Abbildung aller ökonomischen Pflanzen*, Vol. 3, 1789.

If you are in a rage, then the garden can be a mad madder world

Red, seeing

It is not uncommon to see red, what with rage being all the rage. Almost every kind of rage is freely available these days: road rage, air rage, rail rage, political rage, bot rage. In almost every location, there are signs telling us not to rage, but to be kind. However, sometimes, you just see red, don't you? That is when it's time to get into the garden and meet – madder.

This is not madder as in 'Mad Hatter' or 'Mad Max'. There is nothing particularly furious about *Rubia tinctorum* and even the name 'madder' is not what it seems. It comes from the Old English *maedere*, which was the name given to the plant itself, as its roots have been used, more or less since humans started to wear clothes, as a dye. Madder the plant is never going to win any beauty contests, its leaves and stem can be sticky, its flowers are small and yellow, and it grows like a weed. The roots, when washed, are a rather sickly pink and look very much like worms.

Don't judge a plant by its foliage, though, for madder is a plant of kings and pharaohs, of warriors and queens. It was found in Tutankhamun's tomb and has been excavated with Viking material at York. It is madder that was used to create the distinctive red coats of British soldiers from the mid-17th century to the 19th century. Cochineal (from insects) was used for the officers' uniforms, but it was madder for everyone else. Until the mid-19th century, when synthetic dyes were found, it was a mad madder world.

If you are seeing red, you can always go to the garden and find something madder than you are. Or perhaps you can, with some water and mordant (a substance used to fix dye to fabric), make some dye. That could take a while. By the end, you'll be seeing a whole different kind of red.

You feel an overwhelming need for vengeance

Revenge, desire for

Revenge is not one of the seven deadly sins, but that may have been an oversight or, indeed, to do with the fact that the eight deadly sins doesn't have the same ring to it. Still, it's a pretty intense feeling and something to prepare for: the desire to take revenge strikes all of us at some point. The big question is: how? Advice on the best way to seek revenge (served cold) has been around for centuries, but it was never put quite as succinctly as in that great philosophical movie, *Star Trek II: The Wrath of Khan*. (P.S. Wrath is one of the seven deadlies.) 'Do you know the Klingon proverb that tells us that revenge is a dish best served cold,' says the Great Ricardo Montalbán, sucking in his breath before hissing, 'and it's very cold in space.' But who needs intergalactic warfare when you have a garden?

Why not grow a revenge bouquet instead? The slogan goes 'Say it with flowers', and that holds true even if you aren't saying anything nice. But, of course, it's got to be in code. The Victorians loved nothing more than a tussie-mussie, little bouquets that were imbued with meaning according to floriography or the 'language of flowers'. In this arcane, but useful, language, basil means 'hate' and hydrangeas are all about vanity. But, in the spirit of revenge, let's do something a little more sophisticated, not to say passive-aggressive, than just handing over a bunch of moptops.

First, obtain some daffodil bulbs, preferably the later flowering *Narcissus poeticus*, commonly known as pheasant's eye, and plant them up. Narcissi are (in this language) all about egotism and self-love, and so are an essential part of the revenge bouquet. You could then pair them with a scarlet geranium (stupidity) or, to be really spiteful, some basil. Other options include marigold (grief), begonia (a warning), columbine (foolishness), and/or petunia (anger and resentment). Then make the bouquet look very pretty and send it over. Yes, it takes a while to grow a revenge bouquet, but you will feel better immediately.

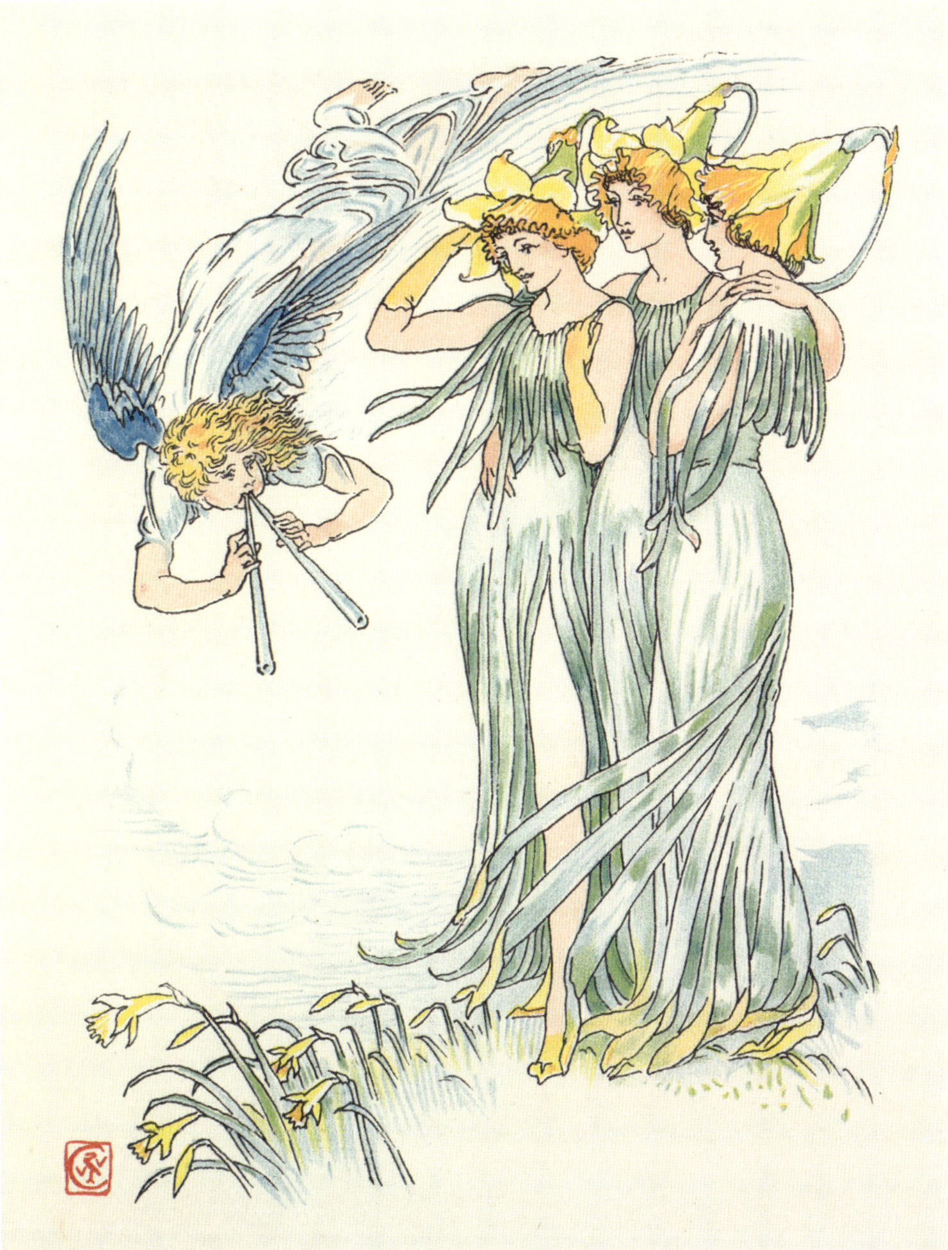

Daffodil figures by Walter Crane, illustrating *The Winter's Tale* in *Flowers from Shakespeare's Garden*, 1906.

Here's a blue-sky strategy for defeating anger

Wrath, all-consuming

The Spanish Roman poet Prudentius (born 348) did a lot of thinking about sin and virtue. In the 5th century, he wrote the allegorical poem *Psychomachia*, which means 'Battle of the Soul'. In it, he depicted the seven virtues as women fighting other women who are the seven sins. The virtues were chastity, faith, good works, concord, sobriety, humility and patience, but it is only the last that we are concerned with here. What strategy did Prudentius use so that Patience could destroy the sin of Wrath? It was all very passive-aggressive. Prudentius donned some serious armour and, refusing to engage, watched as Wrath battled away, crashing her swords into Prudentius to no avail. In the end, Wrath is so furious that she kills herself and Prudentius triumphs.

The garden cure is equally painstaking but manages to avoid large swords and suicidal fury. Imagine that someone has infuriated you to the point where you have lost your grip on reality. You've gone for multiple walks/runs/cycles and are still incandescent. You've bored everyone you know with the details and, finally, you remember Prudentius and decide that the correct strategy is to ignore the entire situation. What you need is to immerse yourself in an endeavour that is both engaging and artistic. We strongly suggest that one such endeavour is *niwaki* or the Japanese art of 'cloud pruning'. This is an exacting practice that transforms a bushy shrub or small tree into an elegant, multistemmed work of art featuring at least seven 'green clouds' at the ends of the branches. All that is required is large amounts of patience and some very sharp secateurs.

There are several options to get started: buy a bush that has already been cloud-pruned or obtain a tiny plant that you then grow and train over a period of many years. The 'instant' cloud prune is cheating because it involves no patience, and growing your own from a tiny wisp is doomed to fail as it requires too much patience. The final, and correct, garden cure option is to transform a young and healthy evergreen bush or small tree. (Ideal specimens are pine, yew, Japanese privet, cotoneaster, laurustinus – but it is worth experimenting with all sorts of evergreen shrubs.)

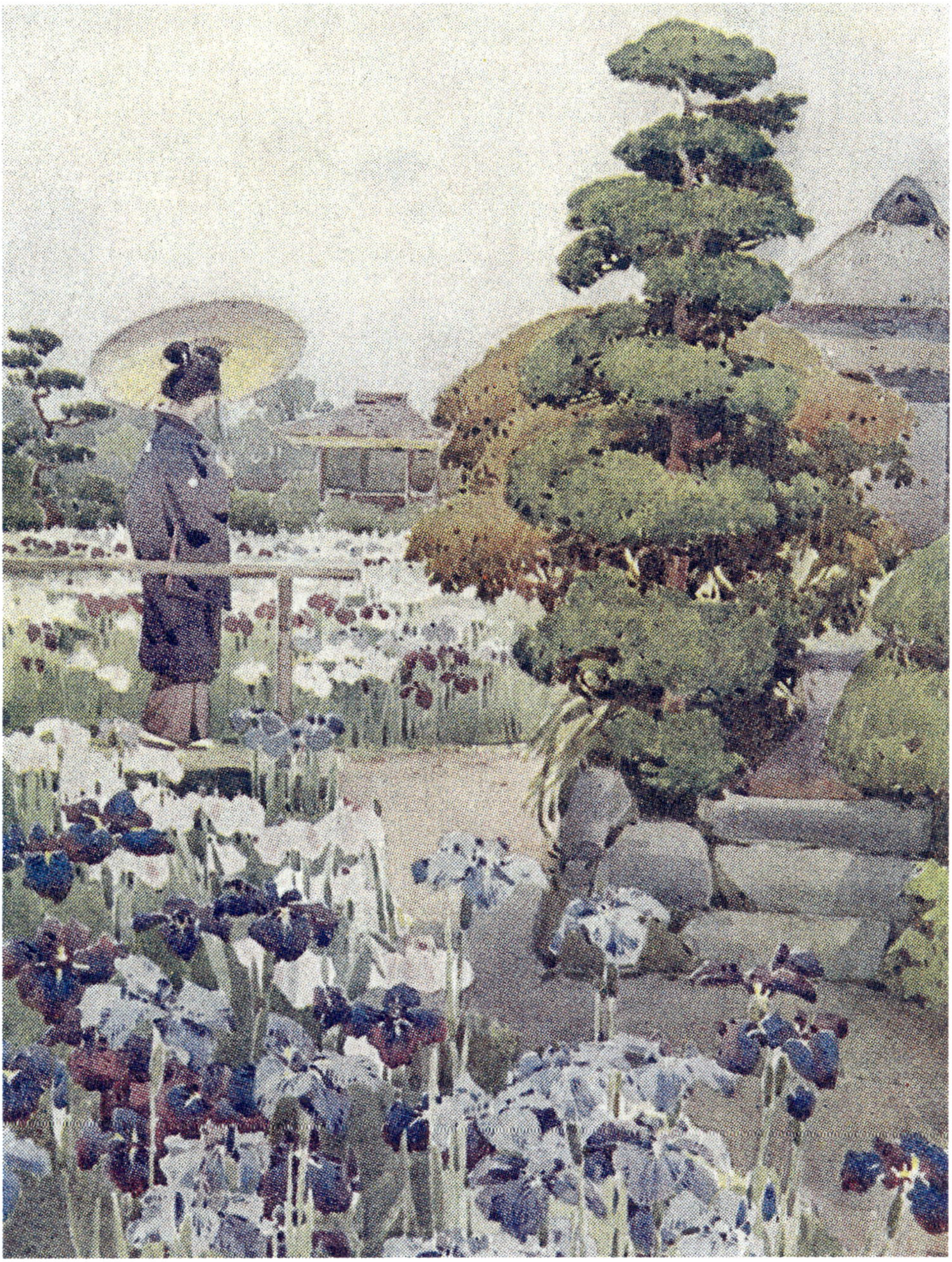

Iris and cloud-pruned tree by Ella Mary Du Cane, from Florence Louisa Du Cane's *The Flowers and Gardens of Japan*, 1908.

By this point, you've almost forgotten that you are furious. Select a shrub with an interesting branch formation. It doesn't have to be symmetrical and is usually more interesting if it isn't. Figure out which branches you want to keep. Remove all the rest, including any little twigs, working out from the centre. You now have at least seven branches. Trim side shoots into 'clouds' towards the end but avoid pruning the tips until the plant has grown to its desired height and width. Deep breath, as this may require some patience (probably at least a year). If it is already the right size, then prune the tips, which will help the cloud shapes bush out. The whole 'bushing out' process can take a while (more patience). You can always stake or manipulate the branches. Give the little clouds a yearly trim in early to late summer or, if it's fast-growing, twice a year. Then step back and admire your work. How pleasing is that sensation? You have created a thing of beauty and, not incidentally, defeated wrath.

It's perfectly fine to snip, snip, snip sometimes

Kleptomania, tendency towards

The great thing about gardening is that taking cuttings – snip, snip, snip – is not always a bad thing. There is no doubt that digging up plants and carting them away is unacceptable. Many gardeners would admit (if given a truth serum) that they have taken a few surreptitious cuttings in their time and lived to tell the tale. It can be hard to resist when you see verbena or a salvia that looks particularly snip-a-ble. Hydrangeas, fuchsias, rosemary, lavenders are all rather tempting, especially if you just happen to have some snippers in your pocket.

But be aware that some people may see this as 'green-collar crime' and to avoid upset – or indeed accusation – there are two basic options. The first is to adopt the same mantra as foragers, which is always ask permission first. The second is to time your request around the correct pruning time, at which point you won't just be taking something but also giving back.

'The great thing about gardening is that taking cuttings – snip, snip, snip – is not always a bad thing.'

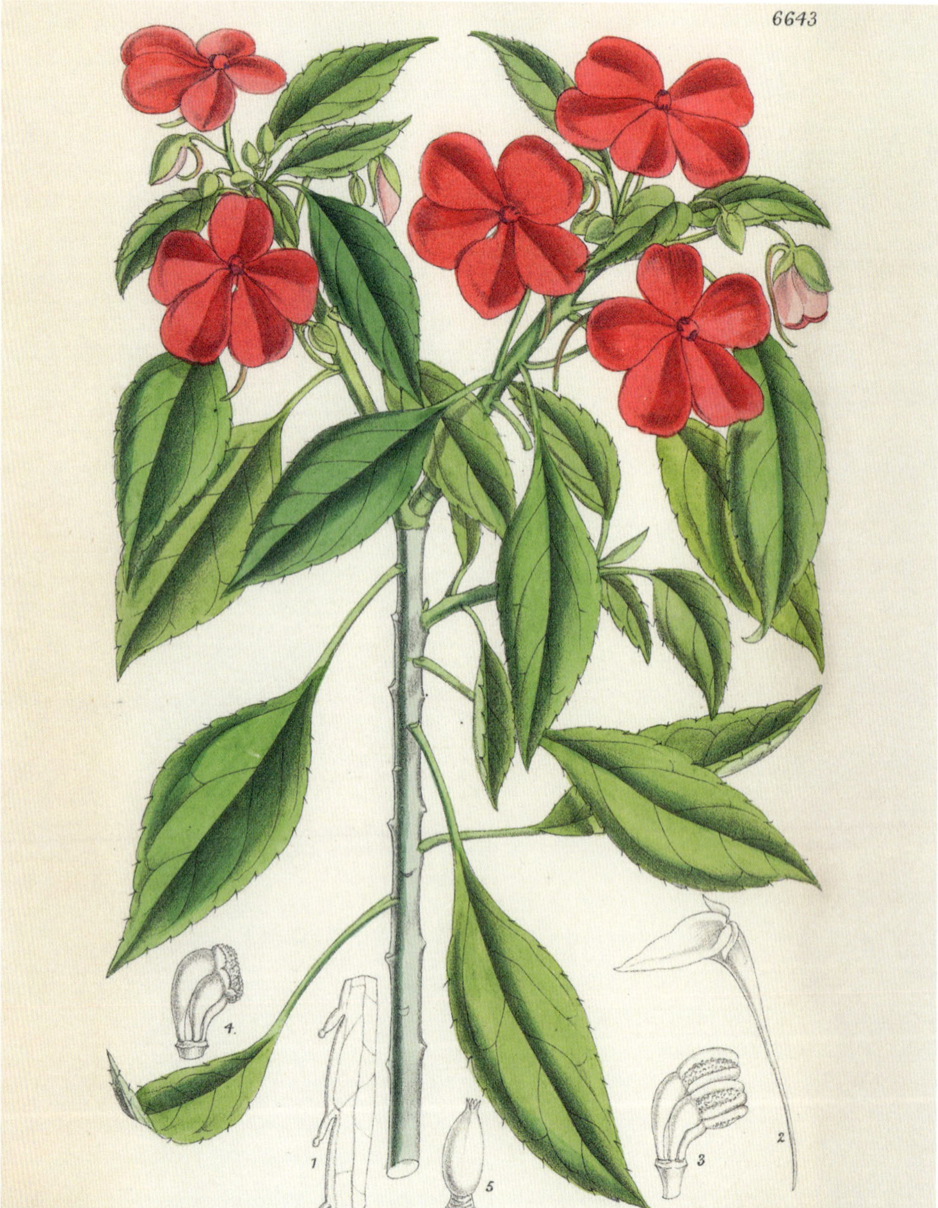

Impatiens sultani, watercolour on vellum (artist unknown), published in *Curtis's Botanical Magazine*, 1882.

There's a lesson to be had from the forever perky Busy Lizzie

Impatience, avoiding

The state of impatience is not easy for anyone to accommodate. It is often accompanied by toe-tapping and tut-tutting, pursed lips and loud sighs. This is why one person's impatience is almost always a shared experience. It's a trait of impatient people that they cannot stop themselves from wanting others to know how they are feeling. It's an ego thing. What they really want is for you to be impatient too. Sometimes it seems as if they are going to explode.

Meet Busy Lizzie. She's impatient too, as in *Impatiens*, which is her genus and means impatient in Latin. She was categorized as such by the father of taxonomy himself, Carl Linnaeus, in 1753. Notice that he did not call her *Occupatus*, which is Latin for busy, even though she is the most diligent flowerer, producing small blooms of pink/red/white/purple all summer long. If Linnaeus was appreciative of her prodigious flowering, he was clearly more impressed by her seed pods, which will explode at the slightest touch, scattering their seeds everywhere. That's the thing about impatience; it trumps so many good qualities.

It's a shame, really, because the plant has an illustrious history. She's native to eastern Africa and the story goes that she was 'discovered' by British plant hunter Dr John Kirk when he was travelling with Dr David Livingstone in Zanzibar, and was named *Impatiens sultani* in honour of the ruler there. Later this was changed to '*walleriana*', a reference to missionary and anti-abolitionist Horace Waller who ended up publishing the story of Livingstone's final days, which included the now infamous phrase 'Dr Livingstone, I presume?'

What's in a name? In the case of Lizzie, quite a lot. Her's has empire and adventure, morality and exploration. But she'll always be known as impatient first. There's a lesson there to learn: if you are impatient, hide it. Then people will see your better qualities first.

Let sweetness into your life

Sourness, overcoming

Let me introduce you to Francesco Cupani. He was a Sicilian, born in 1657 in the village of Mirto in the island's northwest hills. He became a Franciscan monk at the age of 24 and devoted himself to studying natural history and botany, with a particular focus on the island's native flora. Cupani, in addition to having a love of plants, had a definite knack for networking. He either knew the great European botanists of his time – or knew someone who knew them. He was also a prolific writer of letters.

In 1692, he had even more to write about as he became the director of the botanic garden in the town of Misilmeri, near Palermo. Cupani as a writer was not unlike Mount Etna, which he would have known well, bursting with information about his studies of native and exotic plants, sending off seeds in letters, creating herbariums to order. So it shouldn't be a surprise that, in 1699, he sent the seeds of the Sicilian native plant, *Lathyrus odoratus,* to botanist and schoolmaster Robert Uvedale of Enfield in north London.

This is how the sweet pea came to Britain and the original native soon becoming five varieties. Over time, that multiplied, until today, there are at least 1,200. It's a great horticultural tale: how one letter from a Sicilian monk led to such a colourful profusion of this highly scented annual that is now beloved by so many. If you're feeling sour, get your hands on some sweet peas and, for a long-lasting supply, plant up a teepee of them in early spring. Two varieties of note are *L. odoratus* 'Cupani', which is deep purple-blue and maroon, and *L. odoratus* 'Dr Robert Uvedale' with dark purple flowers. Both have a sweet scent that is certain to banish any and all remnants of sourness.

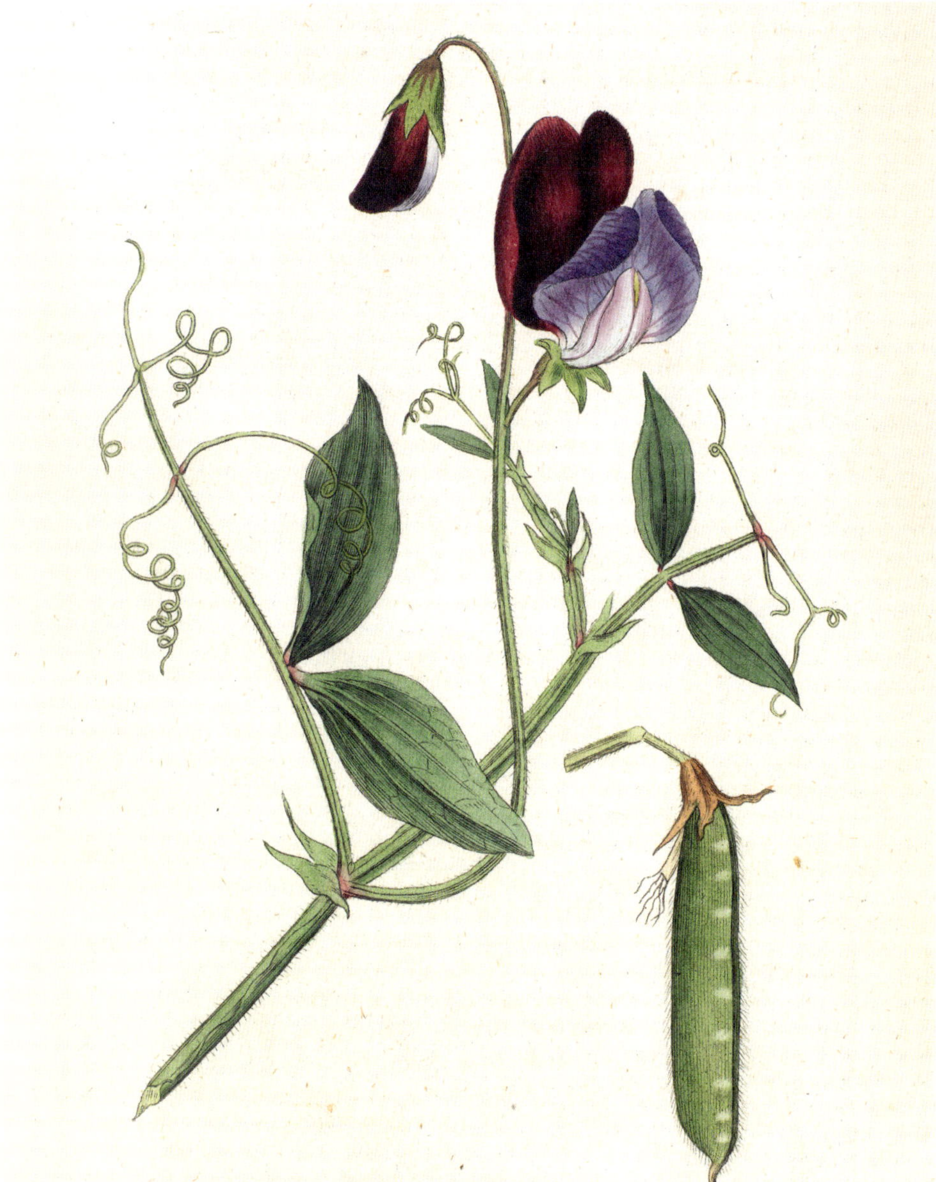

Sweet pea (*Lathyrus odoratus* 'Cupani'), published in *Curtis's Botanical Magazine*, 1788. Artist unknown.

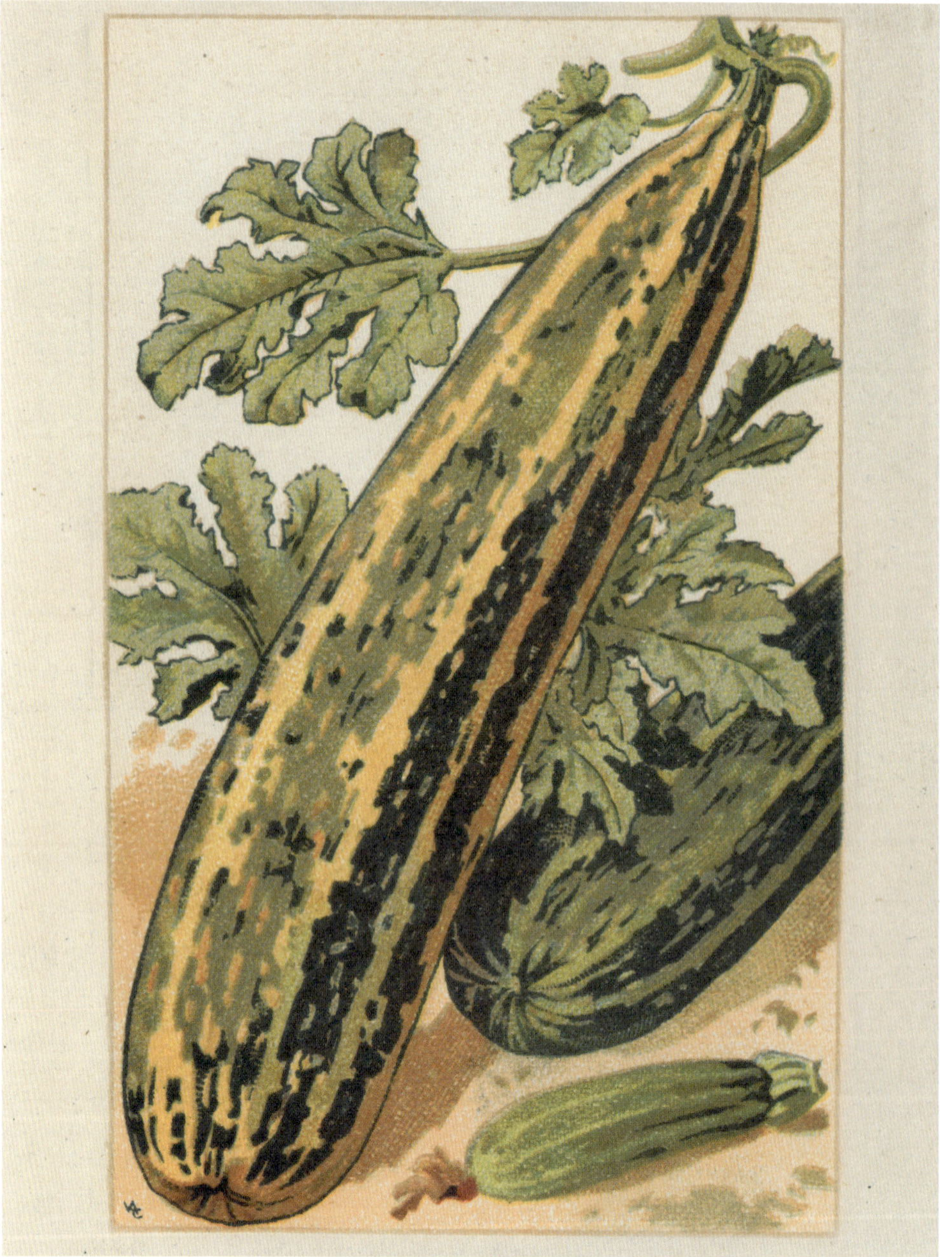

Long green marrow, French seed packet, 1920s–30s.

There's an easy – and cheap – way to experience largesse

Parsimony, habitual

Parsimony, as a quality, has its pluses and minuses. There is nothing wrong with wanting to pay only your part of every bill, down to the last cent (rounding it down if possible). It's when you start to feel you may be tipping over into downright stinginess that you might seek help. There's being careful, and then there's being Scrooge. No one wants friends who are ghosts with chains.

Fortunately, the garden has a cure for this – and it won't cost much either. Buy a packet of courgette seeds. There should be at least 15 in there. Sow about 10 and, of those, choose six to grow. If you are a beginner, then go for the ultra-reliable F1 hybrid 'Defender'. Sow indoors in mid- to late spring or directly outside from late spring. They will start to produce courgettes from midsummer at an average of three to four per week (more in a good year).

This means that, from your six plants, you will have about 24 courgettes a week. Steam and sauté them. Make ratatouille until you can't stand the sight of it. Grate them in salads. Use them in cakes (chocolate courgette cake is an actual thing), muffins, quick breads. Don't forget soup. Give as many as possible to friends and when you run out (of friends) give them to everyone else. Leave them near your gate with a sign that says: 'Free to You' or 'Deliciously FREE'.

Before the end of the season, you will run out of takers and your courgettes will be in danger of becoming marrows. Why not offer them to your local soup kitchens? Or, indeed, anyone or anything? You will be the king or queen of courgettes. You will experience the glow of being generous. You will be a giver, not a taker. One final word: the following year, plant something else. No one wants a million courgettes two years in a row.

Issue a green garden prescription to find a community garden project

Loneliness, feeling of

You can be alone and not lonely. You can be lonely and not alone. Loneliness is a state of being that feels different for everyone and so is hard to describe absolutely. People may feel empty, disconnected, ignored. What's particularly tricky about loneliness is that we often mask it to the extent that sometimes we make ourselves so busy we don't even have the time to clock that, underneath it all, we are seeking a connection we can't find.

Studies show that globally at least a quarter of us have felt, or do feel, fairly or very lonely. In general, loneliness is more prevalent in the young and those in their twenties and it is experienced less by those over 65. It does more than make us feel bad, though. Studies also show that it affects our health, lowering immunity and contributing to raised blood pressure and cholesterol levels. Anxiety and depression can also be part of the mix. Loneliness has been estimated to carry the equivalent health risk as consuming 15 cigarettes daily.

The garden cure comes in many different strands but, in general, studies show that we can feel better mentally just by walking into a green space. The idea that 'vitamin G' is good for us has been recognized officially in the NHS since 2019 when 'green social prescriptions' became available. These usually involve some sort of group activity that can cover a range of activities, including schemes with social and therapeutic horticulturists, but one of the most straightforward ways to fight loneliness is to join a community gardening group.

It's a powerful prescription. In fact, one study by researchers at the University of Essex, tracked people as they worked on community garden projects throughout the Covid-19 pandemic, showing that even in such a deeply stressful time globally, when most others were feeling worse, their levels of health and well-being actually increased. Community gardening groups are easy to find, offering a way to help others and yourself. Another way to dig in, and meet others, is to put your name down for an allotment. Either way, it's a win for you, and for others too.

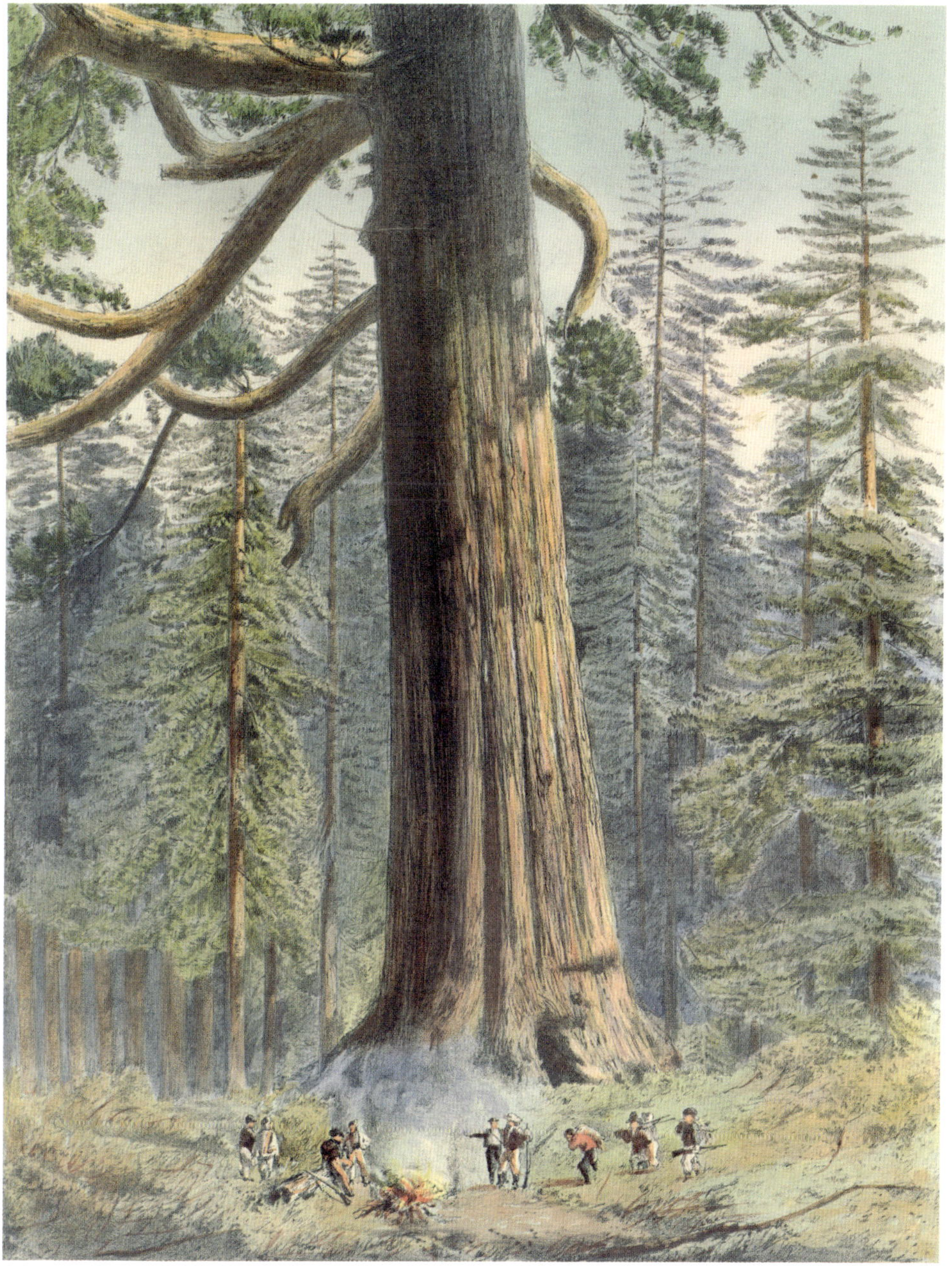

Group outing: giant redwood (*Sequoiadendron giganteum*) by Edward James Ravenscroft, from *The Pinetum Brittanicum*, Vol. 2, 1863–84.

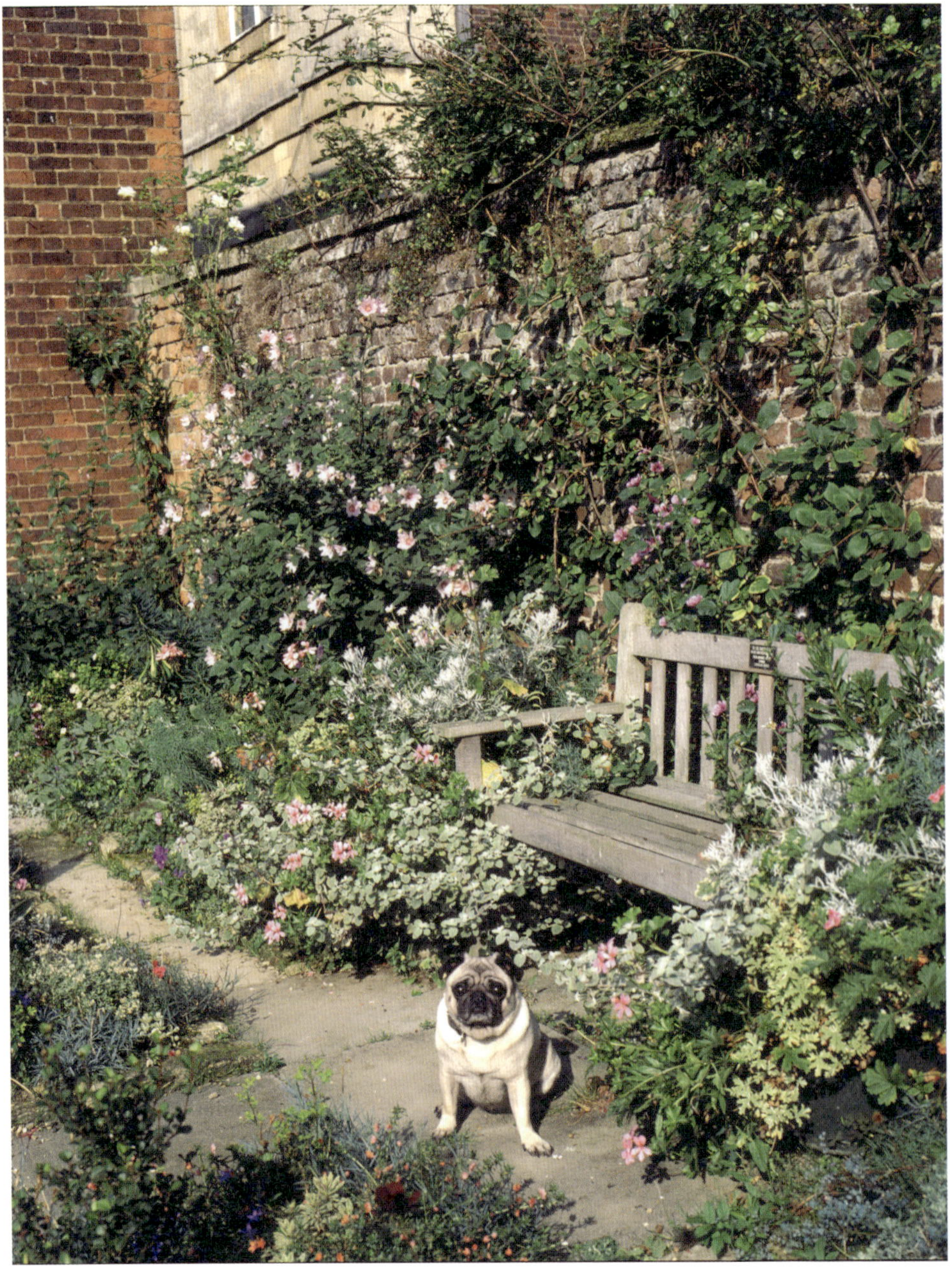

Pug in garden at Dower House on the Boughton House Estate, Northamptonshire, photographed by Valerie Finnis, 1970s.

Dogs and gardens are a win-win

Loneliness, solving

Many famous gardeners have dogs and now, in some cases, the dog(s) have become more famous than their humans. We can probably blame garden superstar Monty Don whose most famous dog was his golden retriever Nigel, who for nine years could be seen 'helping' Don in his garden at Longmeadow in Herefordshire. Don, who has been open about having suffered with depression, credited Nigel with helping him recover. His book *Nigel: My Family and Other Dogs* was a love letter to dogs in general and in particular Nigel who died suddenly in 2020. His next dog, Nellie, died from cancer in 2023. Both are buried in his garden. His current constant companion is Ned. All were (and are) golden retrievers and they receive as much attention, if not more, than their master.

It does seem as if every televised gardener has a pet of some kind nearby as they traipse around their gardens. Cats, who famously choose their owners as opposed to the other way round, never seem quite as dependable (or as helpful) as the dogs, who 'supervise' as they loll about here or there. The dog and gardening theme has become so embedded that Don, along with designer Jamie Butterworth, created a 'Dog Garden' at the 2025 RHS Chelsea Flower Show (where, incidentally, dogs are banned, but that's just because of the human crush there). It featured a lawn which wasn't perfect and various chewed objects, as well as gorgeous perennial planting with paths running through that were 'created' by Ned.

In terms of loneliness, dogs and gardening are a double bonus. Dogs provide loyalty and unswerving love that even your most fervent fern could never quite muster, and the garden makes for the perfect setting for working together. It may indeed be a dog-eat-dog world out there, but, in the garden, it's a perfect companionship. It goes without saying that on TV at least, none of the dogs ever misbehave.

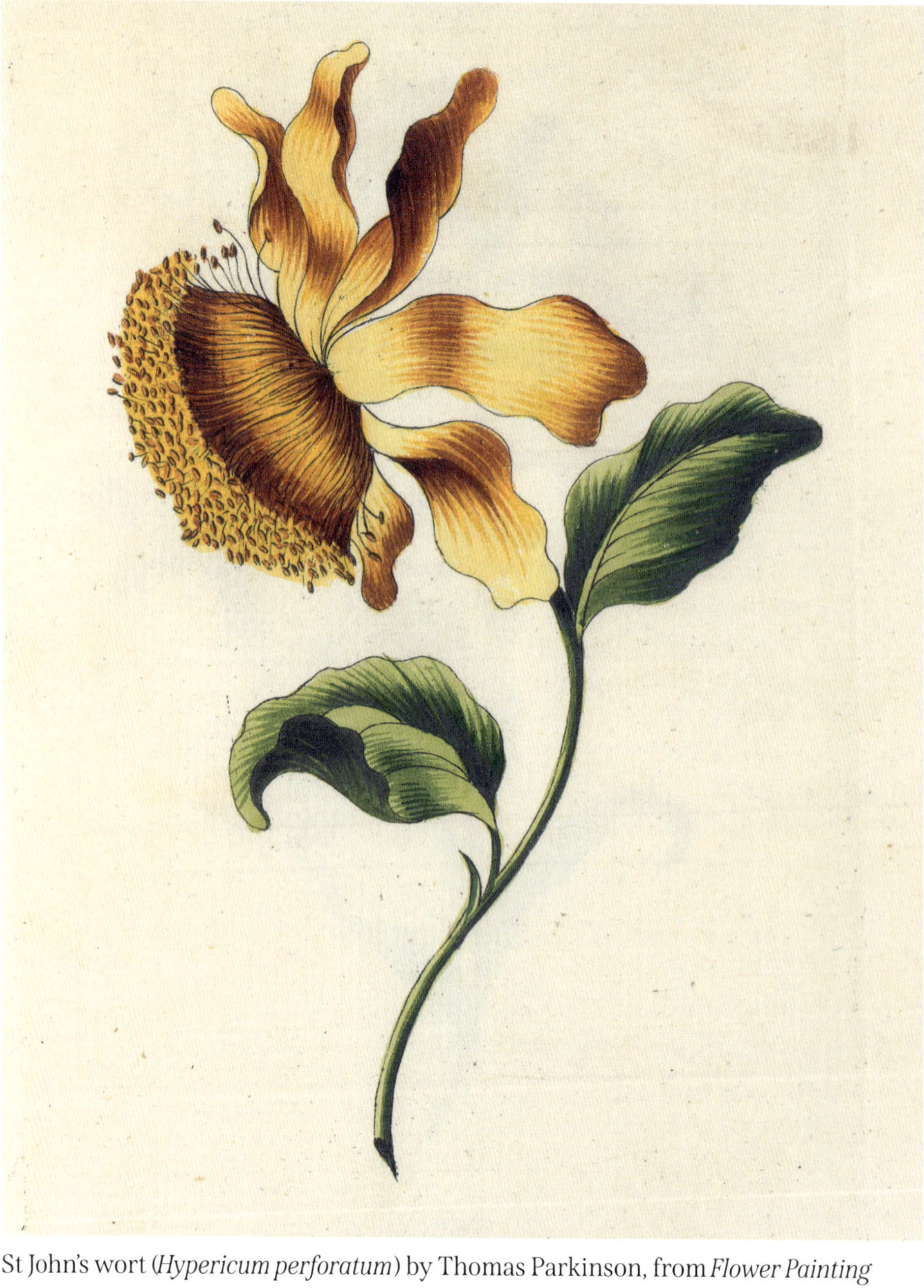

St John's wort (*Hypericum perforatum*) by Thomas Parkinson, from *Flower Painting Made Easy: Being a Collection of Correct Outlines After Nature*, 1760s.

A magical plant of yore rides to the rescue

Mild depression, relief of

St John's wort, the common name for *Hypericum perforatum*, is one of those plants that has a glorious history of magic and power, but which more recently has been seen, in many places, as no more than a weed. In America, it was rampant after being introduced in the late 17th or early 18th century, until its natural enemy the *Chrysolina* beetle was introduced to keep it in check. Quite the comedown for a plant that, from Greek and Roman times through the Middle Ages, was regarded as so powerful that its mere presence was believed enough to instantly banish evil spirits. It is a folklore magnet: supposedly able to protect people from thunderstorms, stop children having nightmares, and cure sciatica and almost everything else. If you trod on it, a fairy horse would appear to charge around with you before leaving you somewhere in the morning, far from home.

There's more (a lot more) of that kind of thing, but then this is a plant that, when you bruise the bright yellow flowers in midsummer, seems to bleed. This is one of the reasons it was seen as magical, being given its common name because it is thought to flower on John the Baptist's birthday (24 June) and bleed on the day of his beheading (29 August). It's not blood at all, of course, but a red oil found in glands in the petal margins.

In the past, one of the many things St John's wort was supposed to help was melancholia, which is one that may carry it through into modern medicine. Studies have shown that it can help with mild to moderate depression. In Europe, it is licensed and widely prescribed for depression, but in other countries, such as the USA, it's only regarded as a herbal remedy, if an increasingly popular one. There are concerns about dosage levels, though, and how it can interact with other drugs. It is thought to work by affecting the levels of certain neurotransmitters in the brain, which results in higher levels of serotonin and dopamine. That is a lot more helpful than a fairy horse.

How a garden of fascination can provide a mental reboot

Lack of focus, overcoming

For many of us, being in our gardens doesn't usually translate into rest and relaxation. We are task driven with holes to dig, seeds to sow, perennials to divide, wisteria to prune. This may indeed provide a way to cope with many of the stresses of life, but it has its limits, and all work and no play doesn't benefit anyone. Riding to the rescue is the work of Rachel and Stephen Kaplan, a husband and wife psychology team from the University of Michigan, who have spent decades researching how we can help gardens help us when it comes to restoring our ability to focus in a world that is full of endless distractions.

Their influential Attention Restoration Theory, or ART, sets out the elements that are essential to a restorative natural environment. It needs to include a sense of immersion, a feeling of being away, and of being at ease with the natural setting. It sounds grand, but all of this can be attained by taking a seat in your garden, even if it's merely a balcony or patio. The final and rather intriguing ingredient is that it needs to include things, such as water or plants, that hold our attention but in an effortless sort of way. Natural flower petal patterns or fractals, for instance, will interest us in an almost meditative way. This state of mind is called 'soft fascination'. These are the four key attributes that will reboot our attention spans.

The idea of a garden of 'soft fascination' is itself fascinating. It should include features that intrigue us in a gentle and undemanding way. A winding path holds our interest more than a straight line of paving stones, though that can be 'blurred' by adding plants that flop over the edges or creepers between the stones. Repeating shapes, such as mounds, will create a feeling of unity and, if used in odd numbers, will hold our attention without trying. A trickle of water (not a crashing waterfall) will catch our eye and naturally become a meditative focal point. Plants that fascinate include those with intriguing leaf patterns and fractal leaf structure (such as ferns) and soft grasses. It's an effortless way to regain control of our mind.

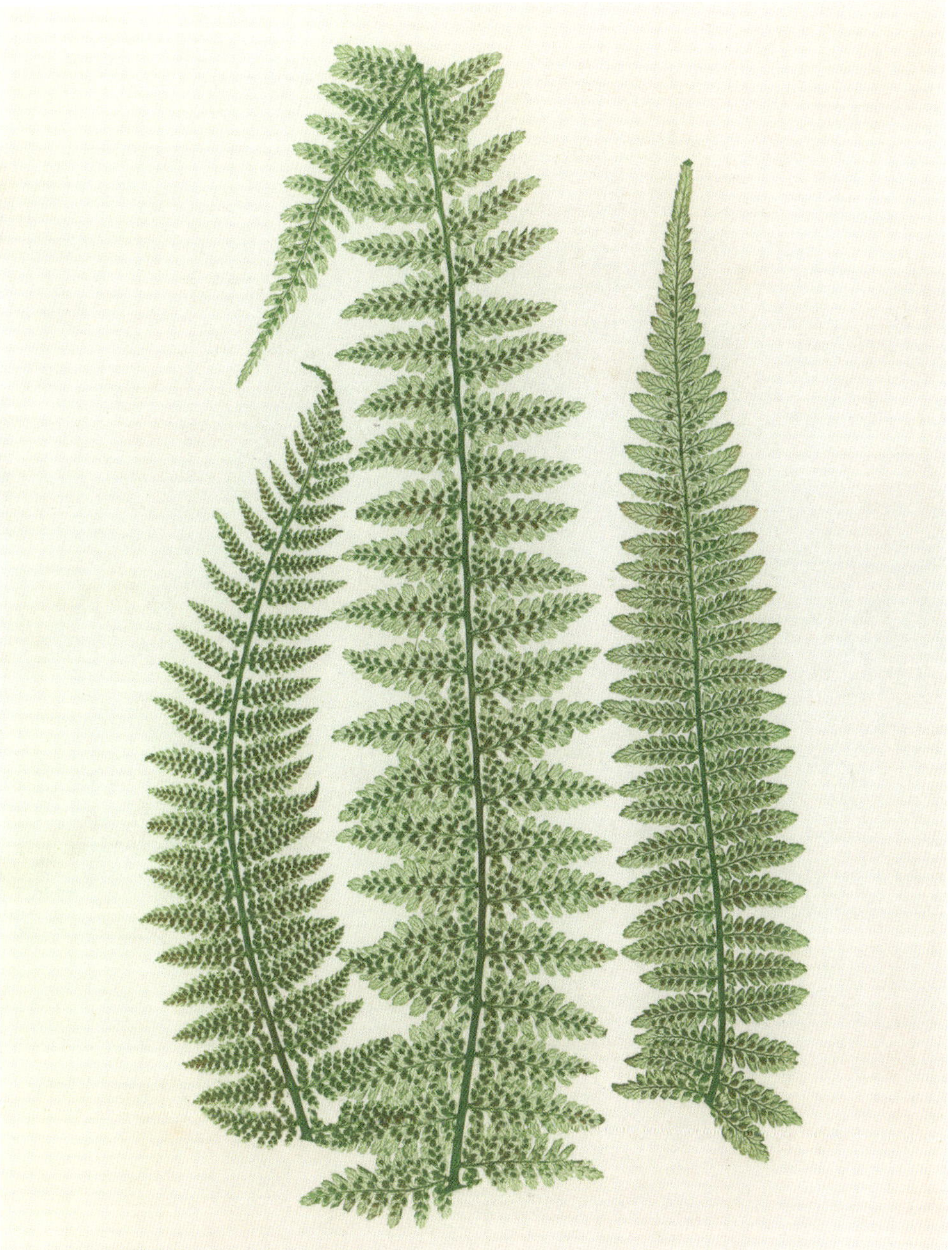

Athyrium filix-femina var. *incisum*, created by nature printer Henry Bradbury, from Thomas Moore's *The Octavo Nature-Printed British Ferns...*, 1859–60.

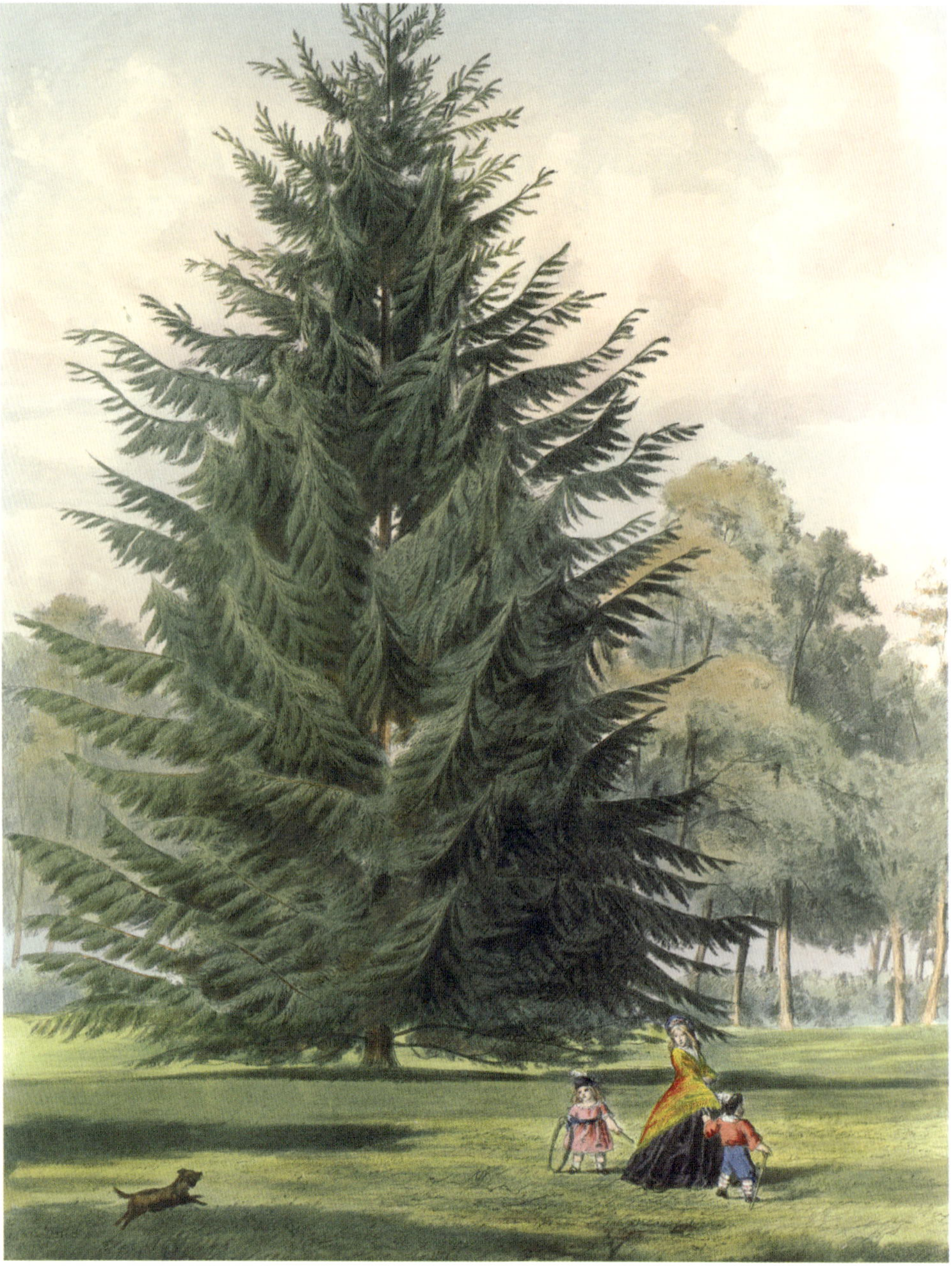

Pinetum scene by William Richardson, from *The Pinetum Britannicum: A Descriptive Account of Hardy Coniferous Trees Cultivated in Great Britain*, Vol. 2, 1864.

It sounds almost too simple but green space is key

Dementia, preventing

Here's an extra reason why we should get outside as much as possible, and that includes for exercising. And yes, the word 'exercise' does encompass the activity that we call gardening, though it could also be running, walking, yoga, hula-hooping, and so on (see *Exercise, Need to Do*, page 17). Studies show that when we are outside our brains are more relaxed and this in turn lowers oxidative stress. This is the stress that leads to cellular imbalances, with free radicals running amok, damaging our cells, which contributes to ageing and age-related diseases such as dementia. The less oxidative stress we have, the longer we live and the better we live. The news that being outside affects this is a game-changer.

The key to this anti-ageing process is an enzyme called telomerase which helps regenerate DNA in our chromosomes and potentially prevent illnesses associated with age. It is found in something called telomeres, which are the protective caps at the ends of the chromosomes found in our cells, preventing damage to the DNA in cells and allowing them to divide without losing genetic data. These telomeres typically shorten as we age and this shortening is associated with age-related diseases. Several studies have shown that being in green spaces slows down the rate of telomere shortening, which results in better health with fewer age-related diseases.

Telomeres are seen as critical biomarkers of ageing and longevity and, though the biology sounds complicated, it boils down to this: being outside, in our gardens or in nature, will help us live longer and better. It gives our brain a rest and a reset. When it comes to dementia, this is all about prevention and that's what green space can help give us.

There's help to be had from a wintry favourite

Alzheimer's disease, managing

The common snowdrop (*Galanthus nivalis*) may look small and delicate, with its slender green leaves and nodding, white, pendent blooms, but it is anything but. All parts of the plant are toxic (no herbivore is going to nibble away at this little one) and it possesses a natural antifreeze that inhibits the ice crystals that kill so many other plants. Plus, its leaves have specially hardened tips that help break through frozen ground. That's quite an armoury for a flower that looks entirely innocent in every way.

Galanthus nivalis is native to central and southern Europe, as well as Turkey and the Caucasus, and is thought to have come to England in the 16th century. It's a common churchyard plant and was grown in abbeys to treat *mal de tête* or 'headache'. There are now thousands of varieties: it's one of those plants that has a sophisticated fan base. Galanthophiles are serious collectors who will pay large sums for unusual or rare bulbs.

It is not known what inspired Russian scientists in the 1940s and 1950s to study *Galanthus woronowii*, a species with broad, bright green leaves, which is native to the Caucasus, and break down its chemical structure. All parts of the plant were found to contain a chemical which they then called galantamine, but it is particularly concentrated in the bulbs. It wasn't until the 1980s that it was discovered that the chemical can be used to manage Alzheimer's disease (the most common form of dementia) as it elevates the levels of the neurotransmitter acetylcholine in the brain. This improves memory and cognitive function and has been shown to be effective in managing early to moderate Alzheimer's. It's also been discovered that galantamine can also be found in other members of the Amaryllidaceae plant family, such as daffodils. The next time you see a snowdrop, give it a nod: it's much more than just a pretty face.

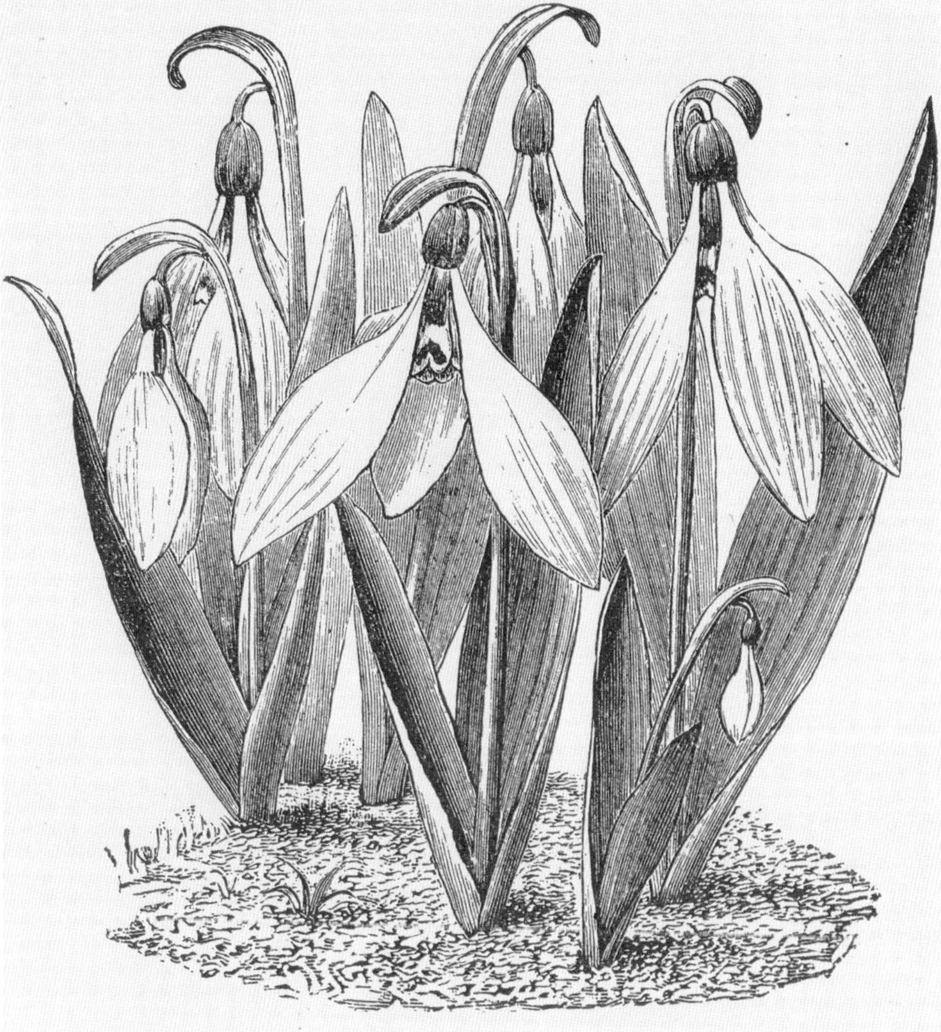

Snowdrops (*Galanthus*), from Dicksons of Chester nursery catalogue *Dutch & Other Flowering Bulbs Etc.*, 1896.

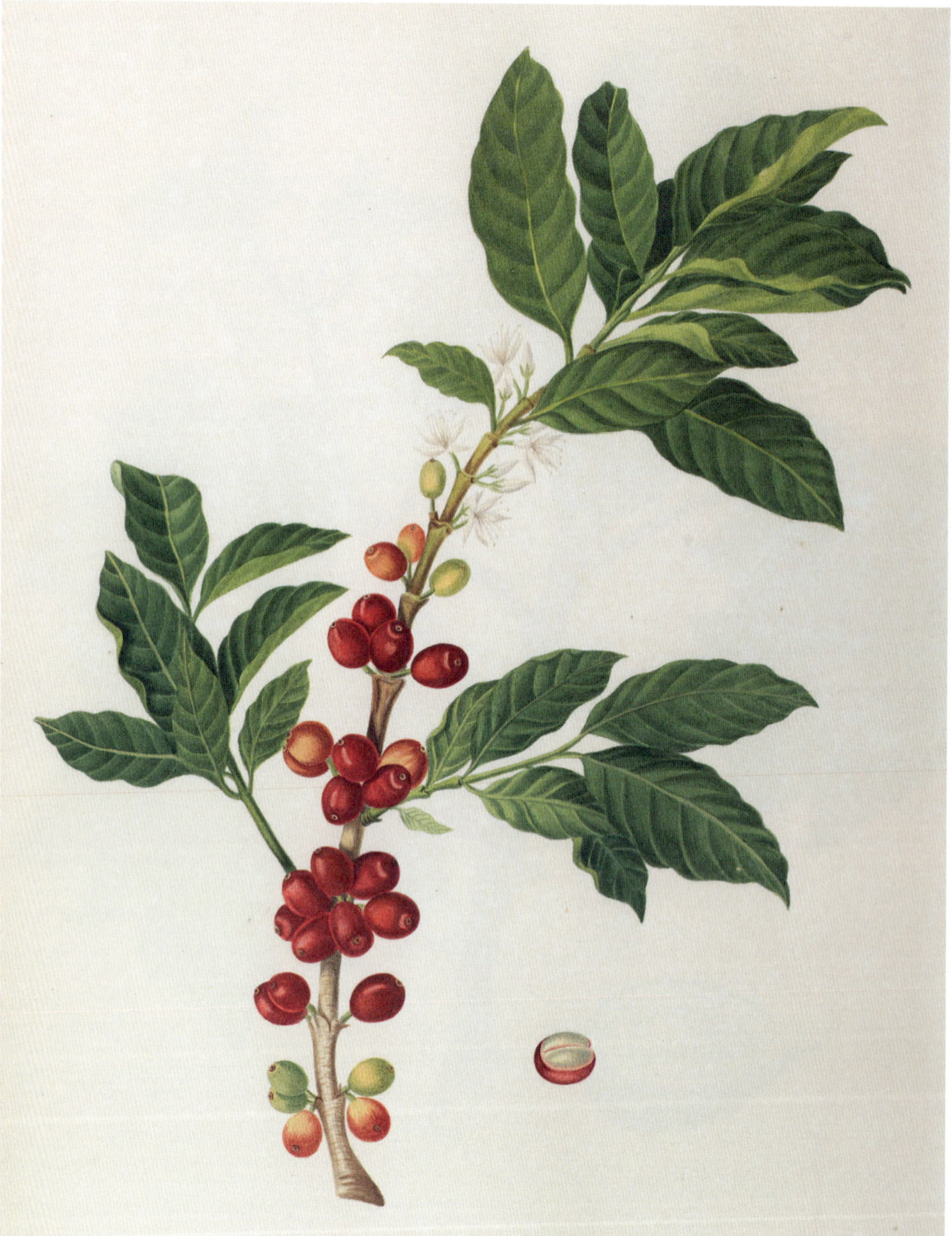

Coffee beans (*Coffea arabica*) painted by Gerrit Schouten, from the album *Schouten Surinam Orchids*, Vol. 2, 1825.

A cup of coffee, even in the sauna, is one answer

Pick me up, needing a buzz

The story of the coffee bean (though it's actually a seed) is a rags to riches tale. It begins in Ethiopia in the 9th century when, legend has it, a goatherder called Kaldi in the Kefa region noticed that his goats seemed turbo-charged after eating some red berries. Instead of relaxing and lounging about in the sun, they were up and at 'em, prancing and dancing. He showed the berries to a passing monk who then dried them and boiled them in water. Thus the first cup of coffee was created.

Coffee was an Arabic drink, popular in Persia, Egypt, Syria, Turkey and Yemen by the end of the 15th century. The first London coffee house followed in 1652 and the rest is Java history. The seeds contain a plant alkaloid or chemical, namely caffeine, which is a central nervous system stimulant. This gives coffee its 'get up and go' energy and is undoubtedly one of the reasons that there are now 2.5 billion cups of coffee drunk globally every day. The countries who drink the most per person are all Nordic, with Finland topping the list. Apparently, though estimates do fluctuate, Finns consume four to eight cups a day and there's a strong tradition (as well as legal obligation) for regular *kahvitauko* or 'coffee breaks'. There's even a word for sauna coffee which is *saunakahvi*.

The bad news for sauna coffee lovers is that eight cups a day is not seen as healthy. About four cups a day, or a total of 400mg of caffeine, is considered the limit. Coffee in moderate doses may do more than charge up your energy levels, as it can also lower the risk of type 2 diabetes and depression. But too much caffeine means having the jitters, plus headaches, high blood pressure and heart issues. Drunk too late in the day it can also interfere with sleep. Still, coffee is so much more than just a drink – it's also an entire social networking tool. As the coffee-crazy Swedes say: 'There's always time for *fika*.' That's nice.

A cup of tea is so often the solution to all problems

Pick me up, taking a break

There are very few problems that can't be ameliorated, if not solved, by a cup of tea. That is certainly the view in Britain and, indeed, most of the world if tea consumption is anything to go by. The top tea-drinkers per person are (in order) Turkey, Ireland, Azerbaijan, the UK and Iran. China and India drink the most tea overall due to their large populations. Only a few countries seem to shy away from tea, notably the USA where most of its (low) tea consumption is of the iced variety. When it comes to caffeine, America reaches for the coffee pot.

Tea is the most consumed beverage in the world, other than water. Globally that's 5 billion cups a day. The good news, in terms of quantity, is that a cup of tea has only 25 per cent as much caffeine as coffee. This means you can drink more without being reduced to a jittering babbler. There is only one plant that is the source for all 'true' teas and that is *Camellia sinensis*. Legend has it that tea was discovered in 2737 BCE when Chinese emperor Shen Nung was sitting under this tree and some leaves drifted into water that was being boiled.

Camellia sinensis has small, white flowers that bloom in autumn and winter, after the main leaf harvest. All of the various types of teas, such as white, green, oolong and black, come from this tree, with their differences created via their processing methods. Tea leaves do contain caffeine, although how much ends up in your cup will depend on the type and brewing method, but they also have L-theanine, an amino acid that creates a calmer alertness, which is different to coffee's wide-eyed hit. This may explain why, so often, tea is seen as something that will calm you down. Shall we have a cup of tea and talk about this more?

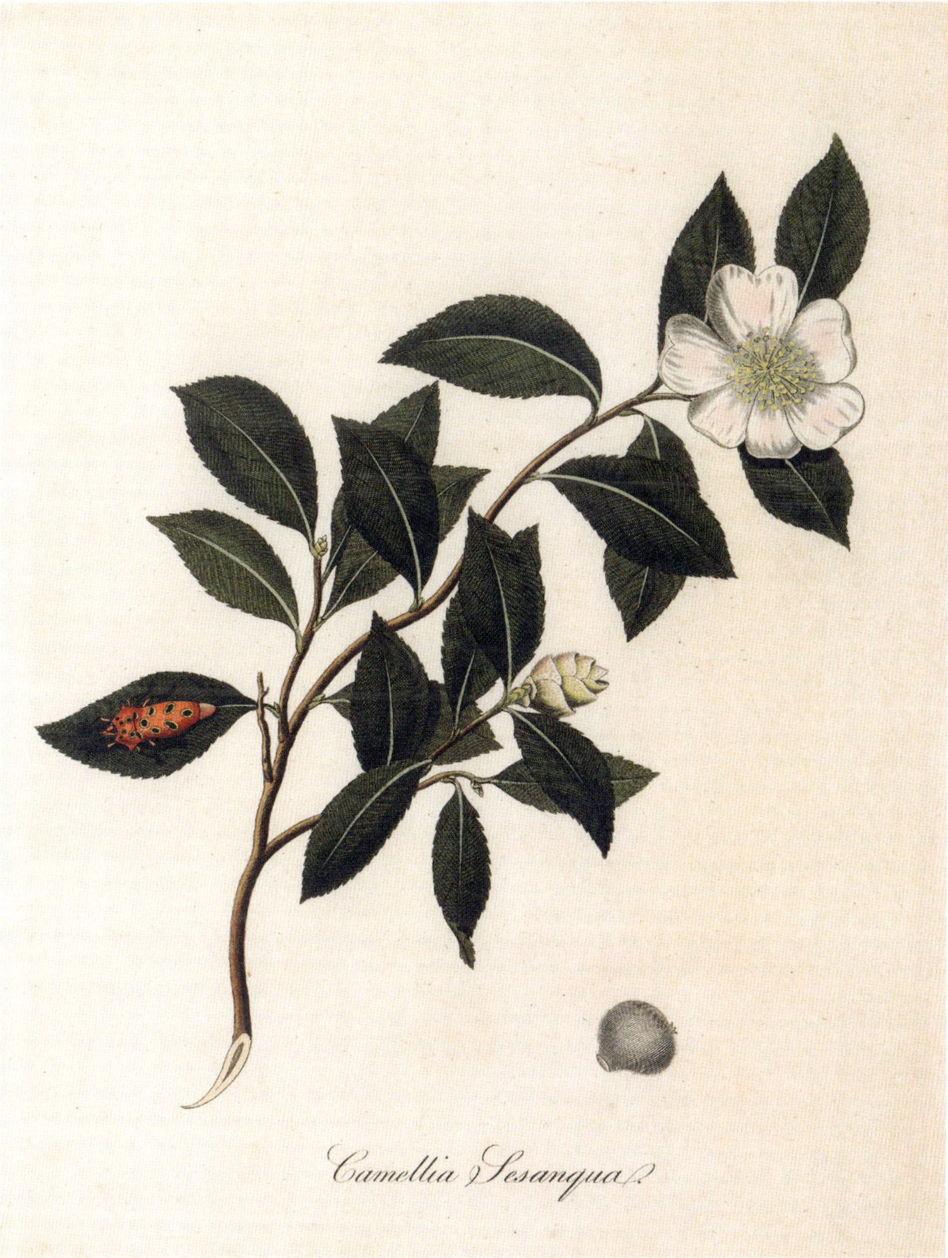

Camellia sasanqua by John Miller (unconfirmed), from John Coakley Lettsom's *The Natural History of the Tea-Tree...*, 1799. This is the prettier cousin of *Camellia sinensis*.

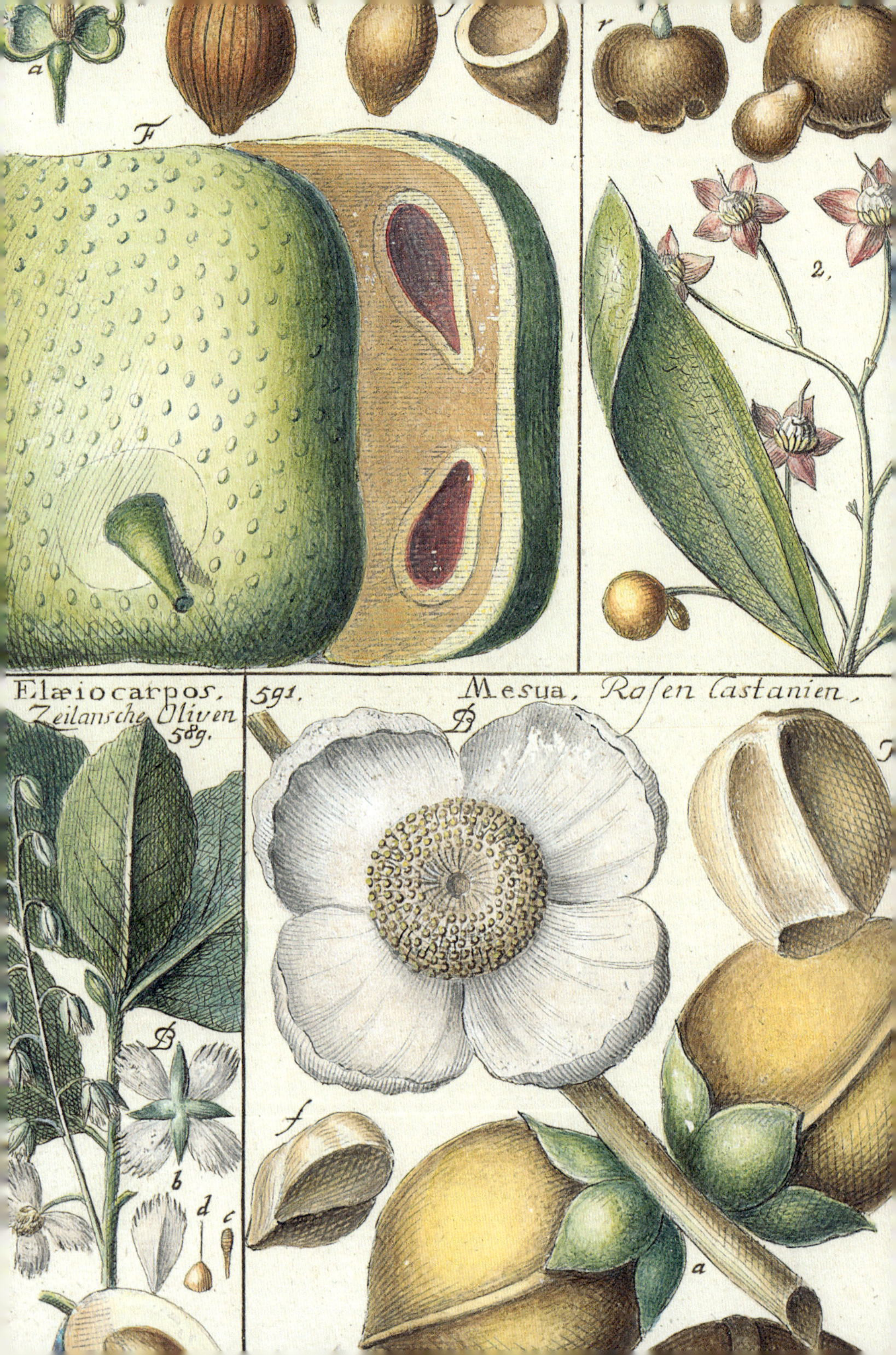
a
F
r
2,
Elæiocarpos,
Zeilansche Oliven
589.
591,
Mesua, Rosen castanien,
b
d
c
f
a

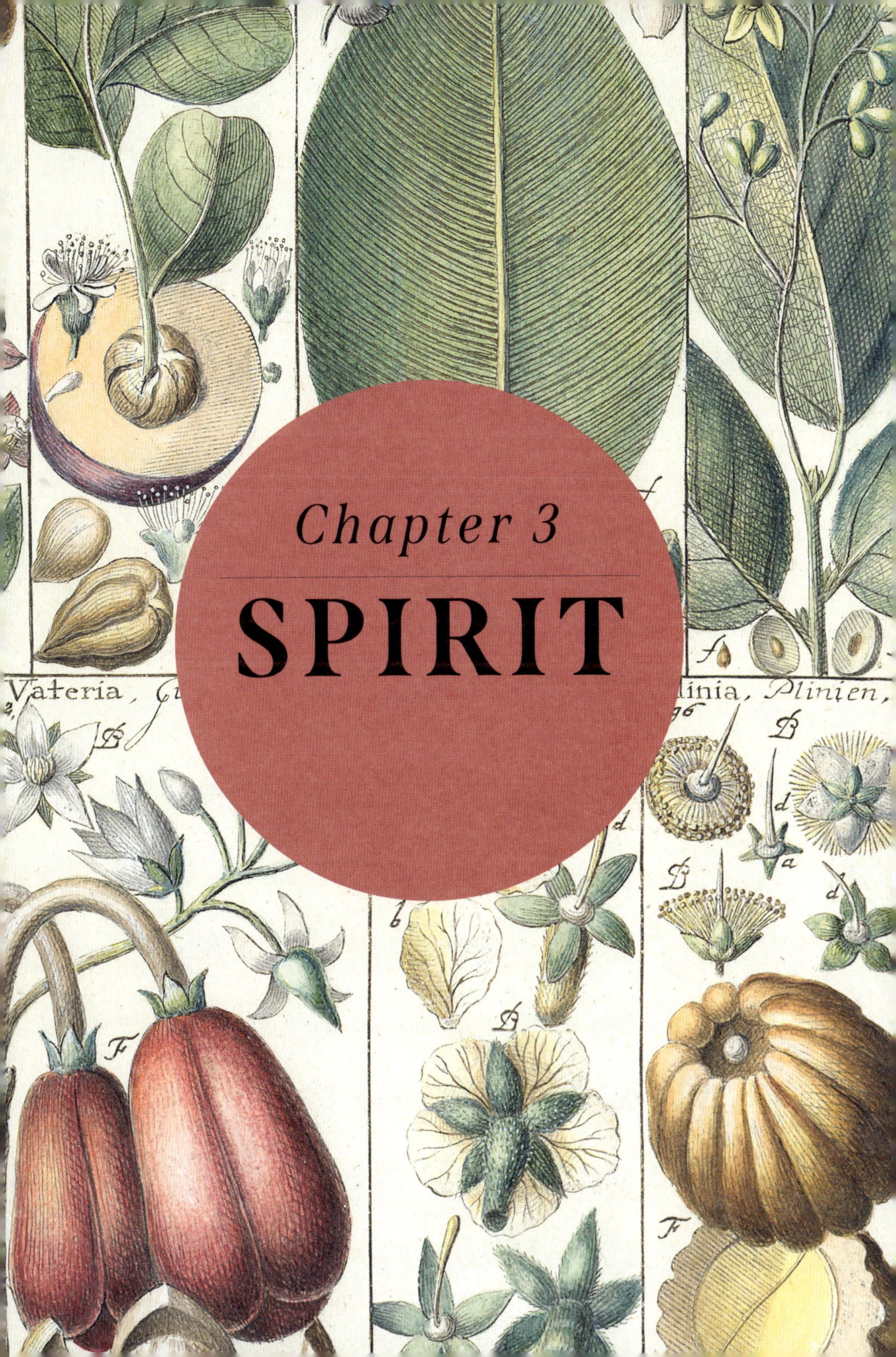

Chapter 3

SPIRIT

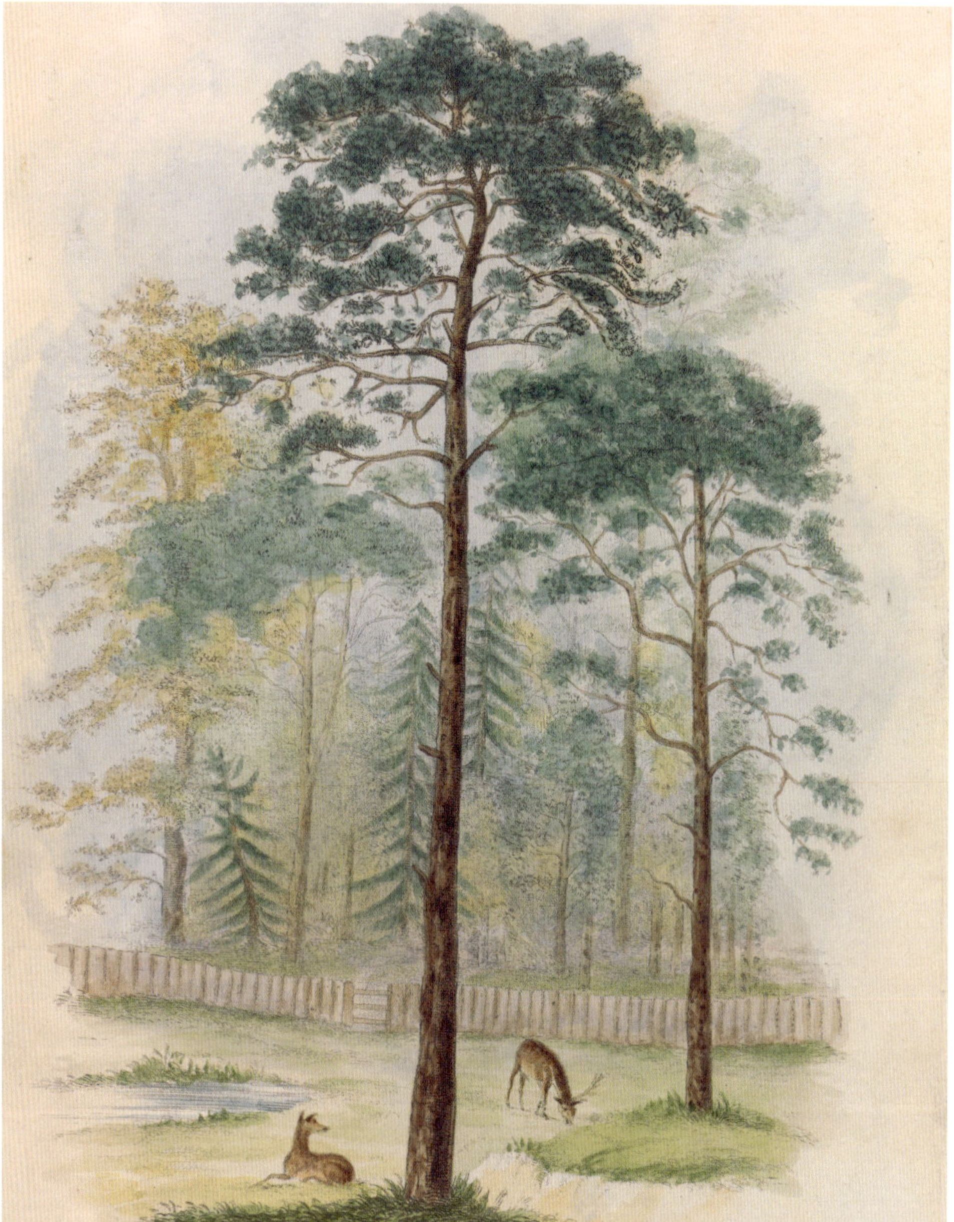

Scots pine (*Pinus sylvestris*) by Ferdinand Lukas Bauer, from Aylmer Bourke Lambert's *A Description of the Genus Pinus...*, 1832.

If you can't live without your phone, go to a forest

Tech-based burnout, tackling

The word 'technostress' was invented in Japan as far back as 1984 to identify unhealthy habits involving what was then called, rather quaintly, 'new technology'. That uneasy feeling that you must be constantly connected and interacting with others has only become more acute. Most of us now spend hours a day on our phones, our brains wired into them, texting, googling, updating, shopping, posting, liking or disliking, watching videos, emailing, Tik-Toking. Cue increased anxiety, depression, insomnia, irritability.

When you are suffering from tech-based burnout you cannot see the forest for the trees in so many ways. It is fitting that in Japan, and increasingly in the West, including the NHS in Britain and in some areas of America, the prescription for this can be found in the actual forest, walking slowly and thoughtfully. Here you are not seeing red (as in anger) but green (as in calm). But you are also activating other senses – hearing the wind and the birdsong, touching the bark, smelling and even tasting the air.

When you are forest bathing, there are no phones or screens of any kind. No tree identification apps. No bird recordings. No endless photographs. This is a no-filter forest experience. Studies in Japan show that this simple prescription has a complex and overwhelmingly positive effect on us: improving anxiety and depression, blood pressure and heart rates, immune systems and sleep. Phytoncides are antimicrobial organic compounds released by plants (particularly conifers) to protect them from insects and bacteria. Now we know that inhaling them is also good for us. And breathe, as they say.

When you can't go to the mountain, make your own

Adventure, lack of

If you are lacking in adventure, then introduce yourself to Sir Frank Crisp. He was born in Suffolk in 1843 and trained as a lawyer (company law) and was given his baronetcy for advising the Liberal Party. So far, so unadventurous, but there was nothing dull about Sir Frank, as epitomized by the garden he created around the neo-Gothic mansion at Friar Park in Henley-upon-Thames, Oxfordshire, which he acquired in 1889. Sir Frank showed the same amount of zeal when it came to gardening as he did the law.

The idea, which was to surround his Gothic monster of a mansion with a 'veritable fairyland' of a garden, was achieved with immense style and pizzazz. Sir Frank welcomed the public in on Wednesdays, and his idiosyncratic guidebook and map includes a Japanese garden, a maze, topiary, a garden of 'sweet smells and savouries' as well as something called 'Nebuchadnezzar's Grass Garden'. There was a rhododendron glen and rose rooteries. The medieval area was comprised of eight gardens, including those edged with wattle and palisades and one called simply 'The Garden of Love'. There was even an area christened 'Ye Vallie of Dancing Downdillies'.

For the more adventuresome there were pools and caves, linked by passages populated by gnomes, frogs, toadstools, swans and nests, including a mysterious item called the 'Nest of Love'. But the main attraction – and the reason that up to 100,000 visitors came from around the world every year – was the 1.6-hectare (4-acre) rock garden inspired by the Alps, a fantasy landscape of huge boulders, pools and waterfalls that cascaded into a waterlily pool.

To create his mountain tableau, Sir Frank brought in 20,000 tonnes of millstone grit boulders from Yorkshire, out of which were fashioned crags and paths, including alpine bridges over precipices. The ambition was breathtaking. There was an Ice Grotto based on the one at Grindelwald and, at its end, an Ice Cave with fake stalactites. But the highlight, in every way, rose above it all at the far end where the (Henley) Matterhorn could be seen. It was some 9–12m (30–40ft) high, its craggy peak a faithful copy of the

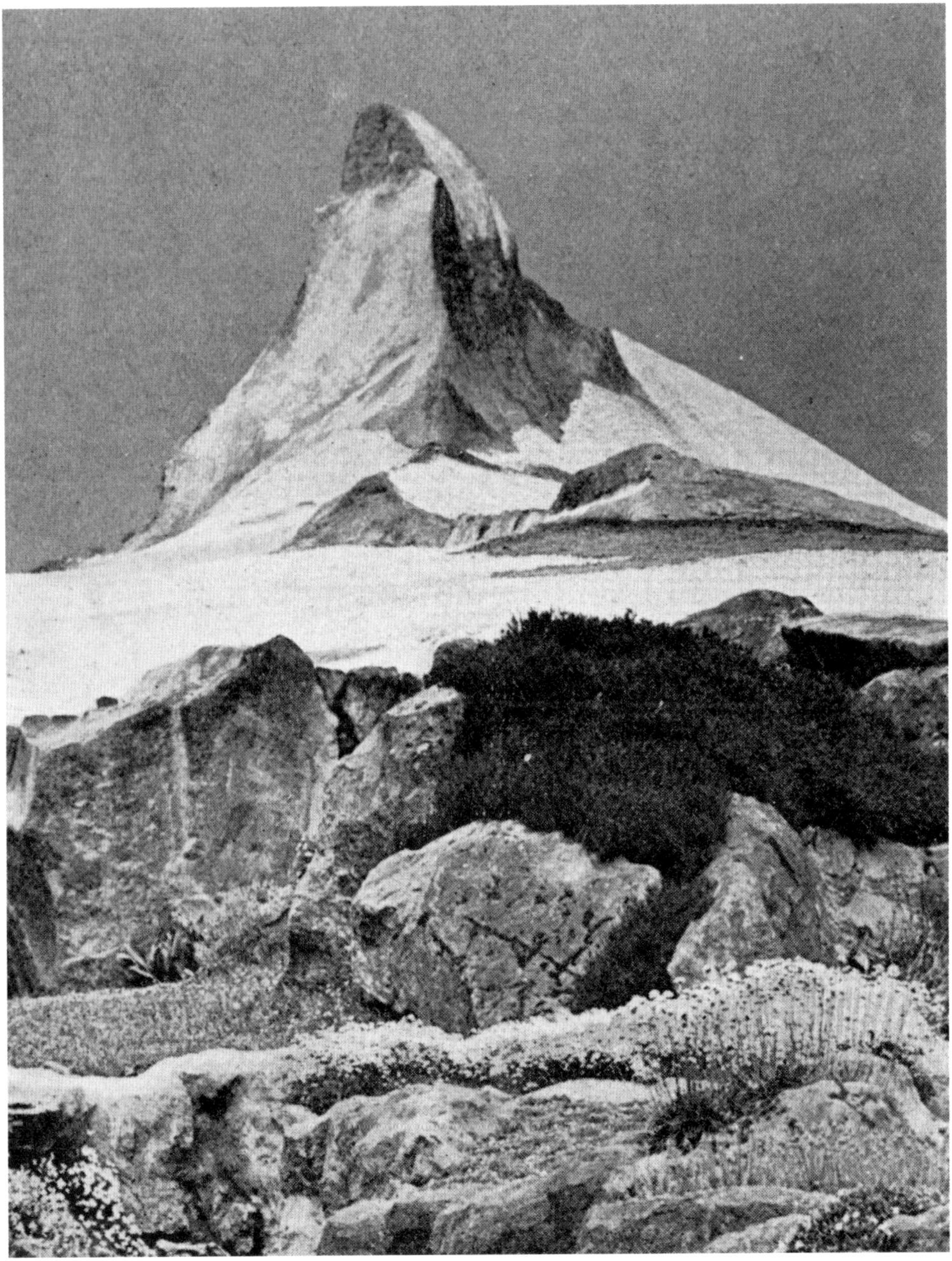

The (Henley) Matterhorn by Frank Crisp, from his *Guide for the Use of Visitors to Friar Park, Henley-on-Thames*, 1914.

original and, indeed, included stone from the original. Derbyshire spar was used to create the illusion of snow. The whole scene was visually calibrated so that visitors, as they meandered the rocky landscape, would have the impression of the snowy peak of the Matterhorn rising in the distance.

The peak, Sir Frank writes in his guidebook, had been fabricated by the head gardener in less than three weeks – what a job to have! Its existence was a huge delight to Sir Frank who, in the guidebook, includes a detailed map of a mock ascent that included the location of the 'Whymper accident' of 1865 on the actual Matterhorn when four men died (their fall is marked with crosses on the garden map). The final 'wildlife' element was added by Sir Frank himself when, as visitors peered at his Matterhorn through a telescope, he would hold in front of the eyepiece some tiny (tin) chamois (goat-like animals) who would appear to be gambolling on the peak.

The planting was no less ambitious. Sir Frank brought in some 4,000 species from all over the world. The result was a global alpine bonanza. Alpinist Henry Correvon wrote, after a visit, how wonderful it was to see natives of the Alps next to those of the Himalayas and Japan and plants from New Zealand challenging those of the Arctic. 'The cacti of Mexico spread their thorns near rhododendrons of our Alps, and the mountain orchids lift modest spikes beside the schizocodon, the famous soldanella of Nippon.'

What an adventure it all was, but the showstopper, in terms of plants, was actually small and delicate. 'Visitors are always astonished to see Edelweiss growing in quite accessible places and with apparently no special arrangements for its comfort,' writes Sir Frank in his guidebook. 'This arises from the popular delusion that the plant requires ice and snow for its proper development, a notion not unnaturally fostered by the Swiss Guides who thereby obtain a higher price for the flower.' There was even an entirely fictional drawing of someone who fell off the mountain, while seeking edelweiss. Very Indiana Jones.

The idea of a garden as a haven is as old as time

Paradise, desire to experience

The word *charbagh* means 'four gardens' and within this idea lies a garden that symbolizes the promised afterlife as described in the *Quran*. This is an ancient concept that can be traced back to 550 BCE and the garden created by Cyrus the Great in his capital Pasargadae in what is now southwest Iran. The land was desert and yet here he made a garden that was both lush and atmospheric. It was walled and divided into four equal parts by paths and rills, all connected by a central source of water. Fruit trees, such as oranges and lemons, provided shade and beauty (and food). Flowers such as roses and lilies were chosen for their scent.

The paradise garden is a formal and reflective space, created to provide a time-out from everyday life and an element of the transcendental. The sounds here are from nature, the rippling of water and the whisper of wind. The flower beds can be raised, sunken or at ground level, but the idea is to be surrounded, as you walk or sit, by beauty and nature. The most famous grand example is the complex covering 17 hectares (42 acres) that is the Taj Mahal of Mughal India in the 1600s. A smaller modern example is the one-acre Le Garden Secret, designed by Tom Stuart Smith in Marrakesh in 2016, with paths of glowing turquoise and beds of flowing grasses.

The paradise blueprint is easy to adapt. You can forgo the rills, dividing the space with paths instead. A central water feature can be a small pool or bubble fountain. The planting scheme can be mostly green or full of colour and scent. Shade can be provided by any number of trees. You'll need some sort of seating, though, to sit and contemplate a world apart.

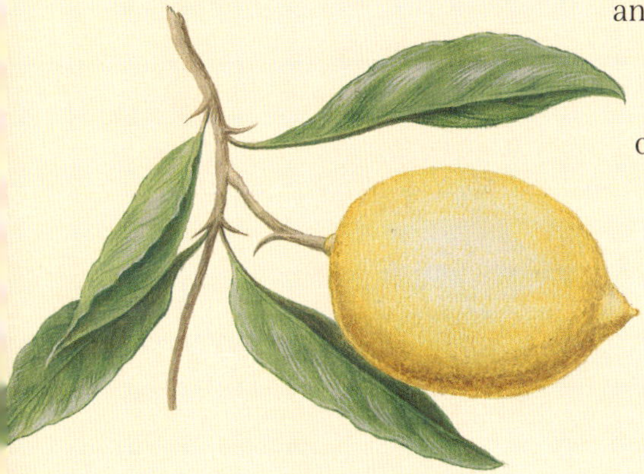

Detail from *Oranges et Citrons*, watercolour on paper (artist unknown), from *Règne Végétal*, Vol. 2, *c*.1800.

When was the last time you felt awe?

Wonder, lack of

Go to Villa Lante, in the medieval village of Bagnaia in Italy, some 80km (50 miles) north of Rome, and stand at the top of the garden, near the grotto, looking out and down on the world. Here, for an entrance fee of a few euros, among statues of the gods and other creatures, you see a garden created by the architect Jacopa Barozzi, better known as Da Vignola. It has been here since 1566 and, somehow, it has been allowed to just be, more or less, as it was created.

The garden at Villa Lante covers some 18 hectares, or 44 acres, and is built on a gentle slope of the Cimini Mountains. It was the newly appointed Bishop of Viterbo, Cardinal Gambara, who commissioned Da Vignola to transform what had been, until then, his 'simple' hunting estate. He created a garden where water is the star, transformed by fountains and rills, pools and cascades, and inhabited by stone statues of creatures, gods and men. Here, there is wildness, but it is contained in a strict order provided by geometry. The central axis of the garden starts at the top, with the grotto, and carries straight down the slope, which has been divided into terraces. There is almost no planting, as we would now see it, or indeed colour other than the green of the tightly pruned hedging.

The overwhelming feeling of unity comes from the restrained planting, with its adjacent woodland feel, and the use of water, which goes from rambunctious to serene, and everything in between, all held within the dark local stone peperino. As you walk down, through Lante, you absorb what novelist Edith Wharton calls 'the ineffable Italian garden-magic'. By the time you finish, it is hard not to be inebriated by it all. The last word here belongs to Wharton, writing in her 1904 book *Italian Villas and Their Gardens*: 'Lante has been exhaustively sketched and photographed, but so perfect is it, so far does it surpass, in beauty, in preservation, and in the quality of garden-magic, all the other great pleasure-houses of Italy, that the student of garden-craft may always find fresh inspiration.' And, indeed, wonder.

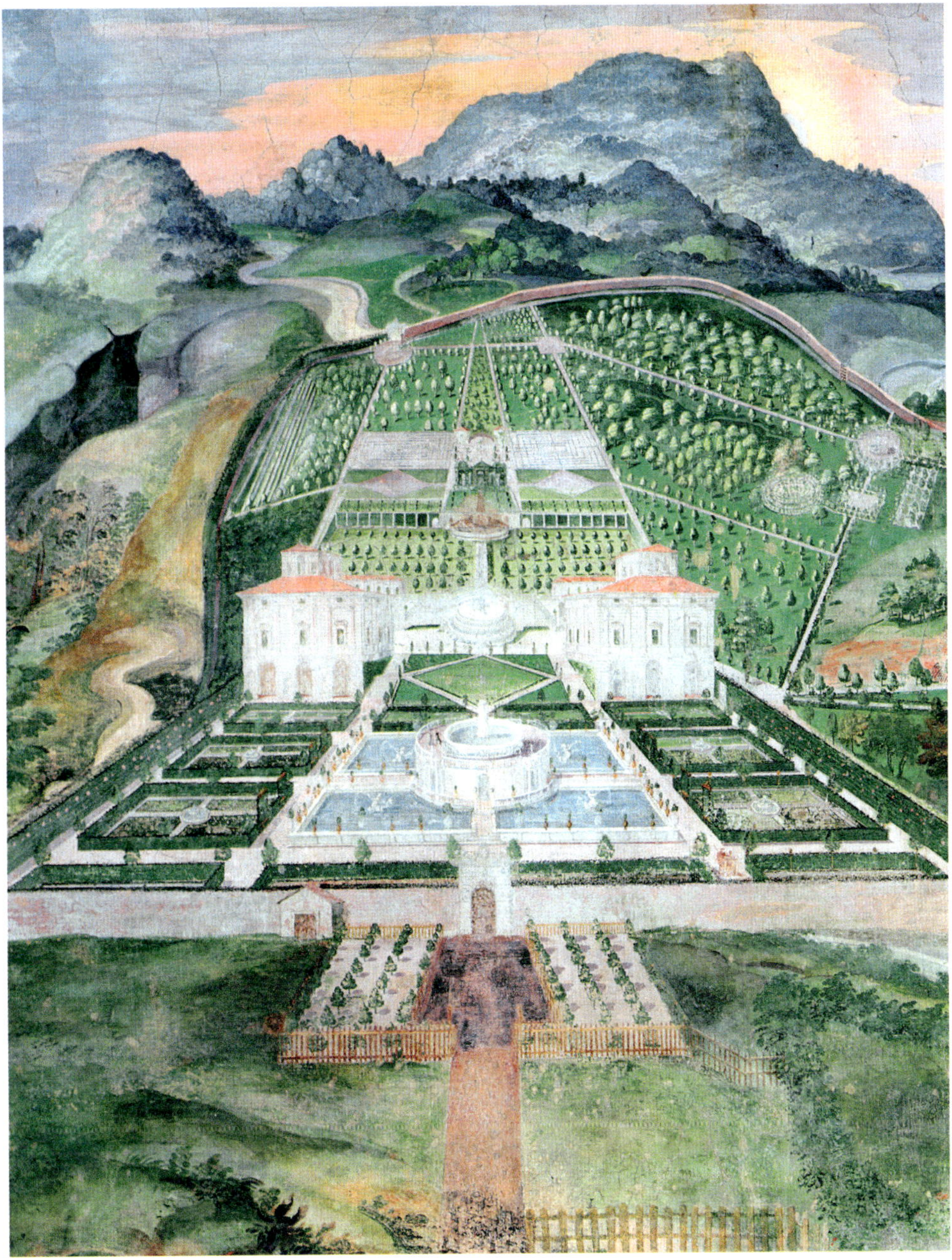

Fresco in the loggia at Villa Lante by Rafaellino da Reggio (Raffaello Motto), 1574–76.

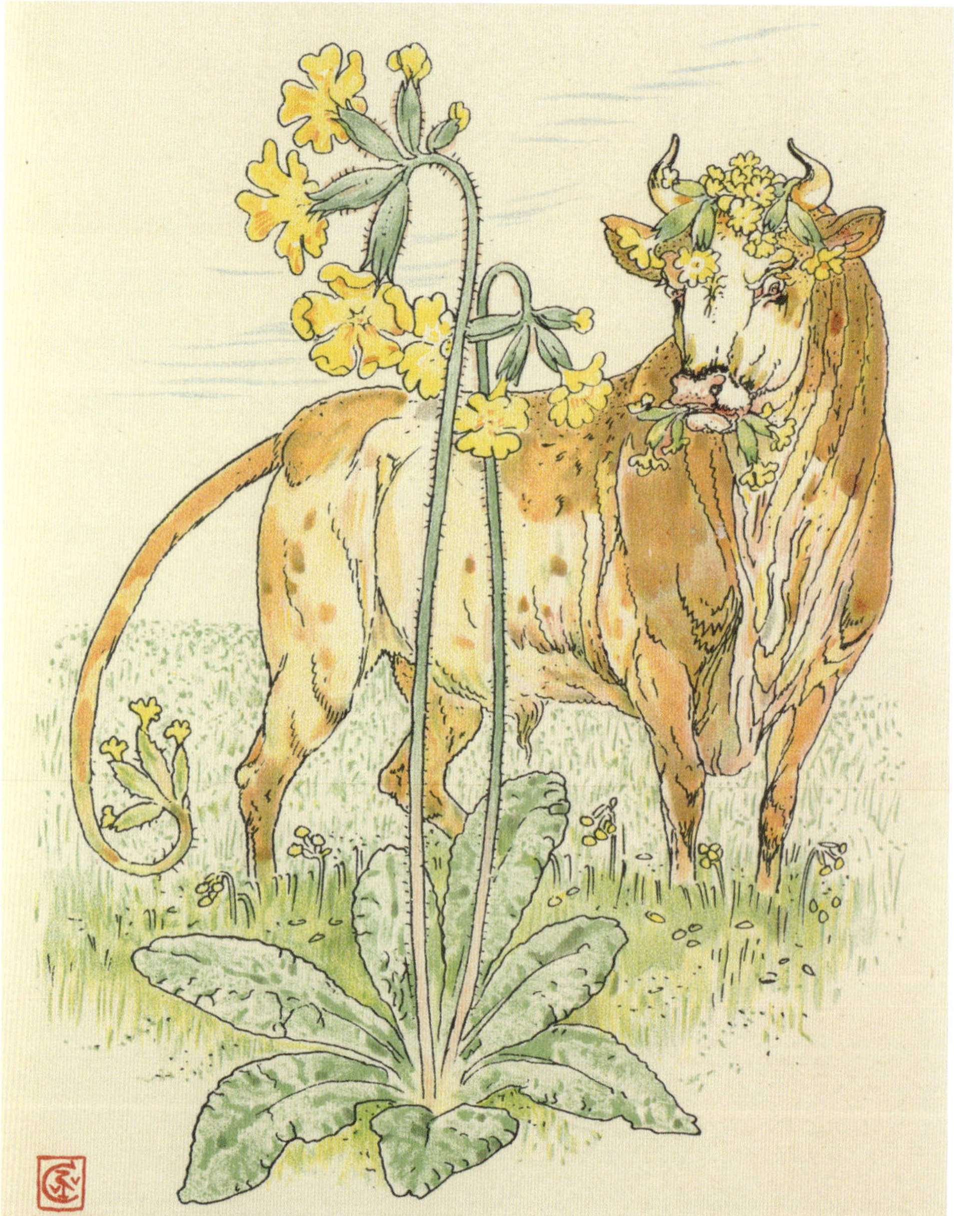

Oxlips (*Primula elatior*) by Walter Crane, illustrating *The Winter's Tale* in *Flowers from Shakespeare's Garden*, 1906.

Let Oberon be your guide to floral luxuriance

Romance (and fairies), shortage of

You do not need to believe in fairies to enjoy their floral arrangements. Shakespeare knew that. There are many of us who have no desire to put up with the antics of the various characters involved in the intricately woven subplots of *A Midsummer Night's Dream*. The King of the Faeries, Oberon, can be particularly irksome, as he plots against Queen Titania, but it must be said that this is one man/king/fairy who can devise a fabulously romantic planting plan, as outlined in this speech to Puck in Act II, Scene I, Lines 249–254:

I know a bank where the wild thyme blows,
Where oxlips and the nodding violet grows,
Quite over-canopied with luscious woodbine,
With sweet musk-roses and with eglantine:
There sleeps Titania sometime of the night,
Lull'd in these flowers with dances and delight.

That sounds like a very dreamy cure for someone who suffers from a lack of romanticism. Why not use Oberon's plan to fashion an arbour, instead of a bank? Create a scented bower intertwined with woodbine (honeysuckle – *Lonicera*) as well as the creamy white musk roses and eglantine or sweet briar (*Rosa rubiginosa*). There can be violets and oxlips below, growing in the shade. Oxlips (*Primula elatior*) are rather unusual and especially pretty, a woodland wildflower with small, creamy yellow flowers, on stalks, all of which grow on one side and look the same way. They are often confused with cowslips (*Primula veris*) or false oxlips (*Primula veris* × *vulgaris*), but only the true oxlip is both one-sided and with flowers all facing one way. Good idea, Oberon.

Look to the Japanese for a poetry in motion

Poetry, lack of

Often it can seem that modern life has no poetry. Sometimes, it feels as if we are living a list as we go about our solitary tasks of shopping online, banking online, texting (online). A theme emerges here. The lack of poetry when it comes to everyday life can be remedied by taking time out to read the fine words of Dickinson or Keats or Auden (and many others), but, in the case of a garden cure, we look to Japan. After all, this is a country that, instead of four seasons, has 72 micro-seasons with evocative names such as Bush Warblers Start Singing in the Mountains (9–11 February); First Peace Blossoms (11–15 March); Crow Dipper Sprouts (2–6 July) and Thunder Ceases (23–27 September).

You could try your hand at creating your own 72 micro-seasons. Don't make it task-based: for example, Prune Wisteria (11–13 February) or Weed Gravel (could be almost any time of year). Observe your garden with all your senses to see seasons such as Blue Tits Start Singing, First Snowdrops Open, Sunflowers Look Upward, and so on. This is a great warm-up when it comes to poetry and the garden. Who needs Andrew Marvell when you can write your own? Actually, we all need Andrew Marvell's *The Garden*, which includes these wonderful lines:

The nectarine and curious peach
Into my hands themselves do reach;
Stumbling on melons, as I pass,
Insnar'd with flow'rs, I fall on grass.

But back to Japan, because that is the land of haiku and that feels more approachable. A haiku is a short poem of 17 syllables arranged over three lines as 5, 7, 5. It usually doesn't rhyme. It's all about capturing a moment in time. Here is a translation of possibly the most famous haiku about a garden, known as the *Old or Ancient Pond*, written by haiku master Matsuo Basho in 1686:

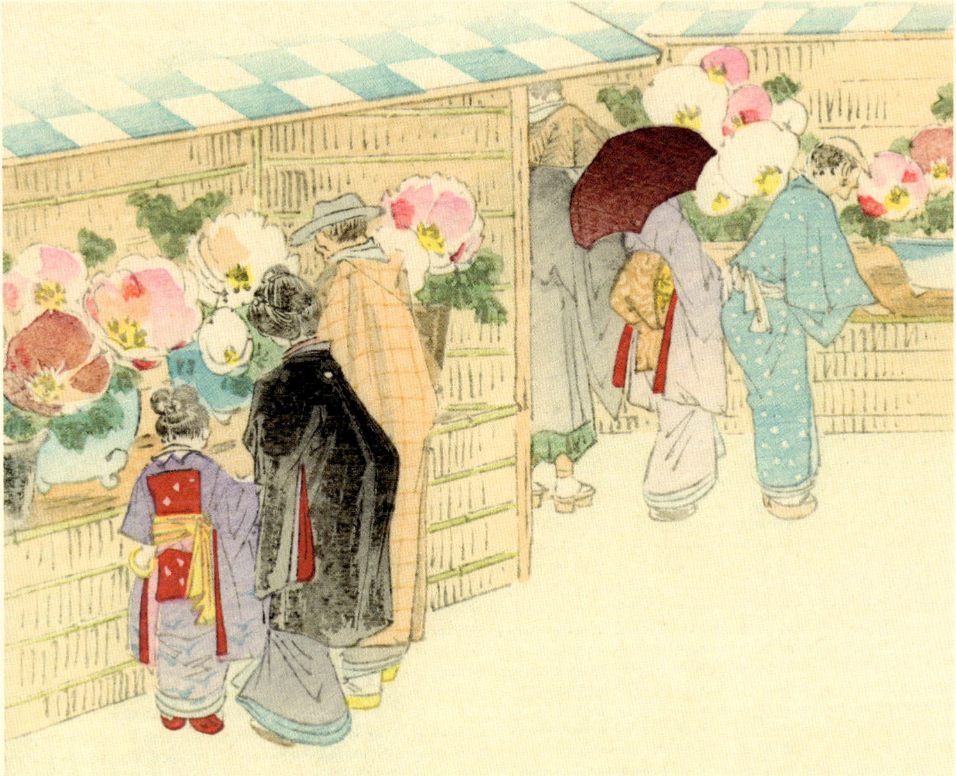

Scene with a peony display from the catalogue of the Yokohama Nursery of Boehmer and Company, 1882.

An ancient pond!
With a sound from the water
Of the frog as it plunges in.

This example is a translation by William George Ashton, so the syllable count is not exact, but it is still admirably succinct and evocative. You can hear the splash – and see the ripples as they move across the pond. Poetry in motion.

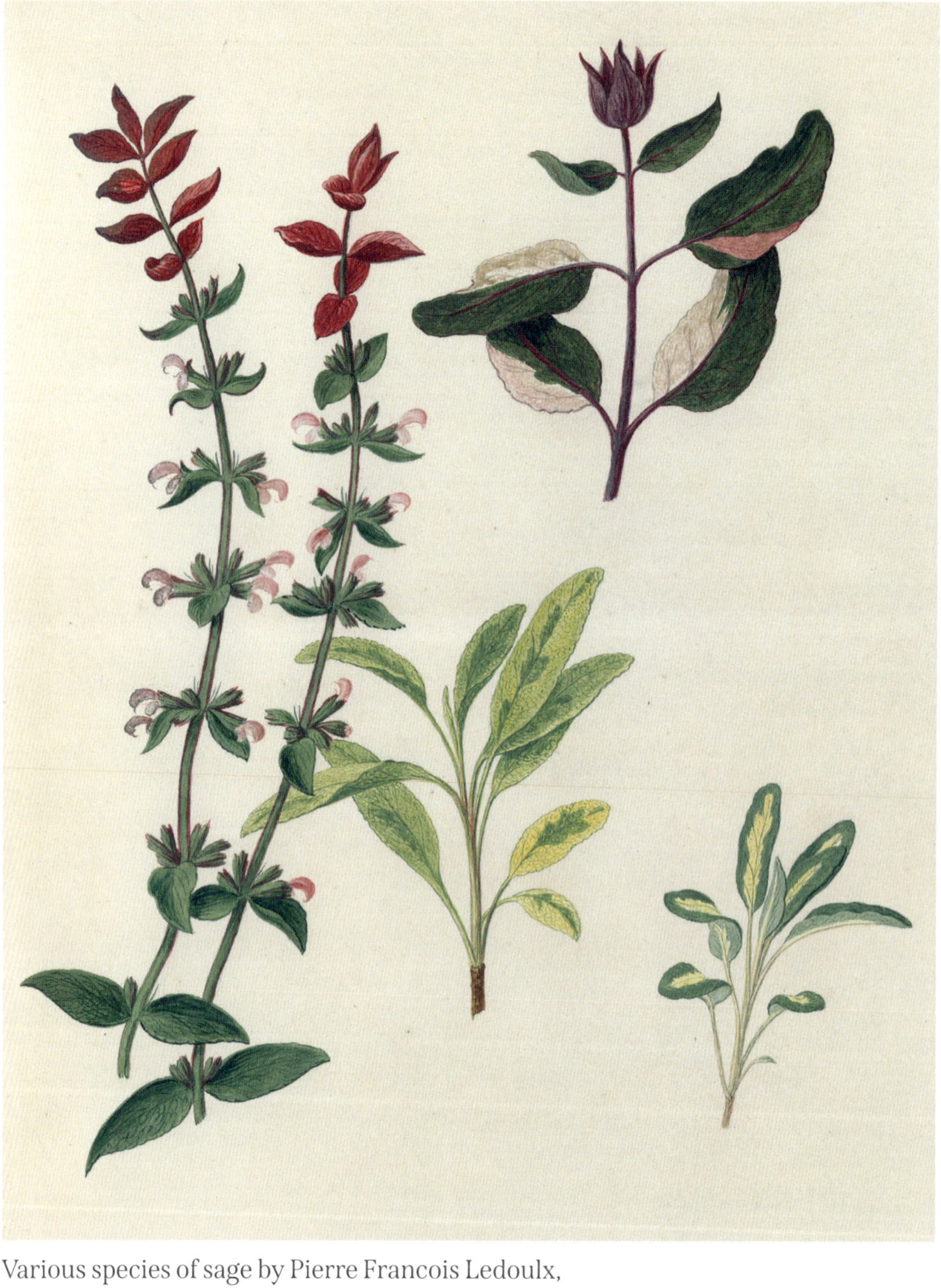

Various species of sage by Pierre Francois Ledoulx, from the album *Règne Végétal*, Vol. 1, *c*.1800.

Smudging with sage is one way to clear the air

Negative energy, too much

Sage is a super-herb that is high in antioxidants and makes a great food stuffing. You can also have it as a tea or fresh or dried with dishes. It is touted as having many health benefits, though studies are mixed and research continues into whether it improves oral health and brain function and lowers blood sugar. But there's another reason to use sage, as a 'smudger'. Smudging is a cleansing practice, aimed at getting rid of negative energy from a space. It was first used by some Native American tribes and has become more mainstream, with sage smudge bundles now sold in a wide variety of stores and health shops.

It's not all spiritual knowledge here. A study showed that burning sage with other medicinal herbs produces major antimicrobial results, reducing airborne bacteria by up to 94 per cent after an hour. It's not the fire that cleanses, it's the smoke. Bee sage (*Salvia apiana*), or California white sage as it is sometimes known, is the favourite, but garden sage can also be used. The idea is to light one end of the sage bundle and then allow it to smoulder. You can be as woo-woo as you like with this, setting intentions, visualizing negative energy leaving the room or house, and even organizing your own cleansing soundtrack to accompany you as you waft. Or you can just do it.

You can cleanse a room or an entire house. Some people smudge when they move into or out of a home, or after a divorce or a major argument or fight. Ideally, the space should be relatively clean and all phones, TVs and electronics turned off. Start at the bottom of the house and move up into the top rooms. In every room, begin in one corner and move around slowly, spreading the smoke throughout, focusing on corners, doorways and windows (which should be open, unless the weather is terrible). You could also use sage to cleanse yourself, smudging it around your body, though, please, no loose clothing. Key final advice: when finished, place the smudge bundle in a fireproof container and let it burn out.

Here's a story that will raise your spirits

Feelings of despair, overcoming

Vita Sackville-West had a talent for many things: writing and poetry, gardening and, indeed, celebrity. She was dubbed the 'bestselling bisexual baroness' after her famed affair with Virginia Woolf, but her legacy is the magical garden that is Sissinghurst in Kent. She created it with her husband, Harold Nicolson, from the 1930s: he did the structure (the hedges are a thing of beauty) and she did most of the planting. In addition to everything else, she was the gardening correspondent for *The Observer* newspaper.

Her column of 22 January, 1950, should be required reading for those who are all too well acquainted with the slough of despond. It begins perkily enough. 'It is amusing to make a one-colour garden,' she writes, adding that if one colour sounds too monotonous, then try for two or three instead as long as 'the colours are happily married, which is sometimes easier of achievement in the vegetable than in the human world.' She says that she is trying to make a grey, green and white garden but that she has her doubts. 'This is an experiment which I ardently hope may be successful, though I doubt it. One's best ideas seldom play up in practice to one's expectations, especially in gardening, where everything looks so well on paper and in the catalogues but fails so lamentably in fulfilment after you have tucked your plants into the soil. Still, one hopes.'

She paints a picture of her future garden, as seen from a rough wooden seat that, in her mind's eye, will be placed with its back against a tall yew hedge. She imagines that there will be low clumps of grey/silvery foliage, pierced with tall, white flowers. The trumpets of *Lilium regale* will be emerging from the greys of the southernwood (*Artemisia abrotanum*), other silvery artemisia, and cotton lavender (*Santolina chamaecyparissus*). There will be white pansies and peonies and white irises with grey leaves. 'At least I hope there will be all those things. I don't want to boast in advance about my grey, green and white garden. It may be a terrible failure.'

Remember this story when you think that there is no hope for something you want. This was a crazy dream of a garden, as visualized by Sackville-West on a cold winter's day in 1950, in a country that had in no way recovered yet

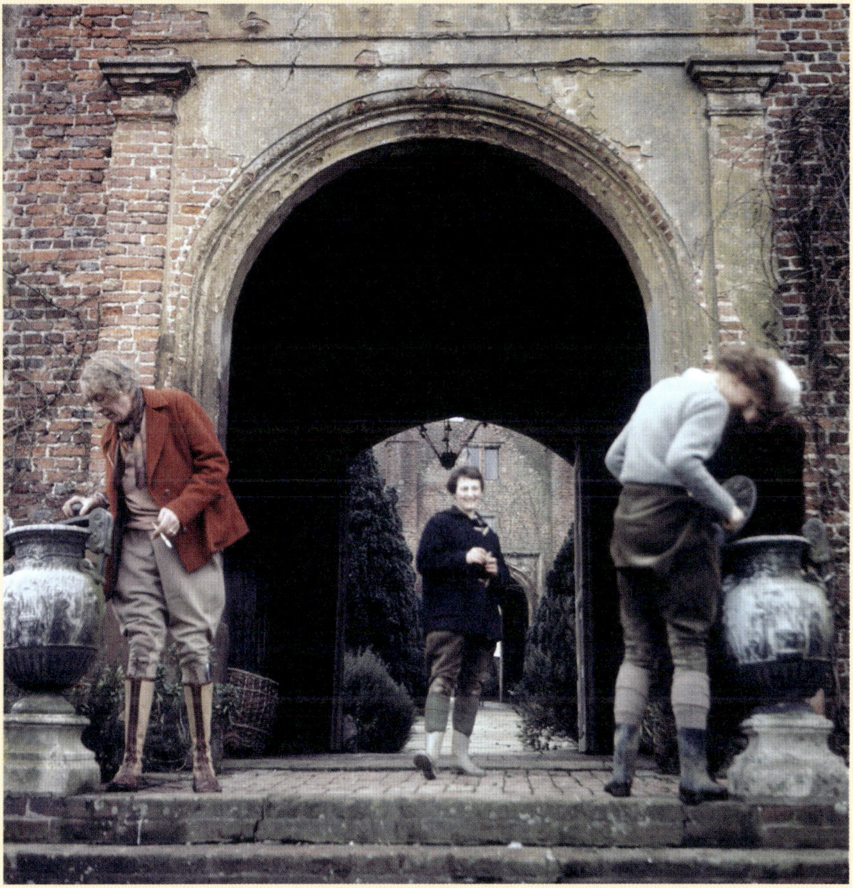

Vita Sackville-West (in red) and head gardeners Pamela Schwerdt and Sybil Kreutzberger at Sissinghurst, photographed by Valerie Finnis in the 1950s.

from the Second World War. Yet despite all her doubts she could not stop herself from hoping that her dream could become something she could see, touch and smell. 'I cannot help hoping that the great ghostly barn-owl will sweep silently across a pale garden, next summer, in the twilight – the pale garden that I am now planting, under the first flakes of snow.' The doubts were real. The fear of 'terrible failure' is imbued in every line of this piece. She had no idea there was no need for all that anxiety. The White Garden at Sissinghurst now is arguably one of the most famous gardens in the world.

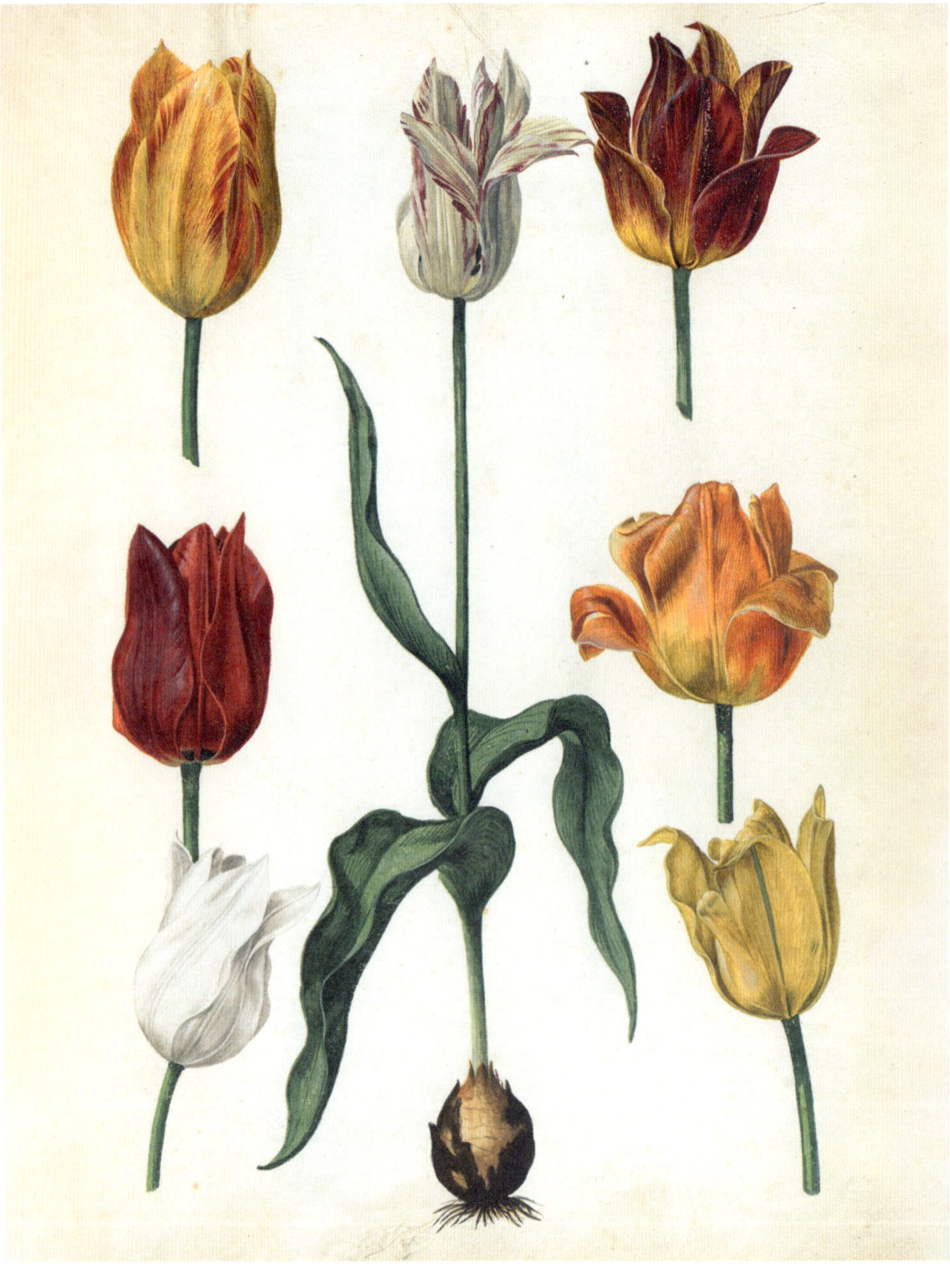

Tulip cultivars, watercolour on paper by Pieter van Kouwenhoorn from his album of paintings, 1630s.

If you feel there's something missing in your life...

Humdrum life, unhappy with

You may not be able to pin down, exactly, what the problem is. Perhaps it's just an uneasy feeling that there should be more to life than this. Maybe your days have become all too predictable: awake, breakfast, work, lunch, work, home, dinner, TV. That's all work and no play. Remember that no one ever said on their death bed: 'I wish I'd finished that spreadsheet a few hours earlier, so that everyone would have been more impressed.'

The garden has a cure for this because it has been known for a garden also to become humdrum. Sometimes, it's just a little dull when your garden is so low maintenance that it contains only work-a-day plants that require virtually no maintenance. No wisteria (too demanding). No climbing roses (ditto). No espalier apples (double ditto). You know the gardens I mean: nice but no cigar.

What's missing? In gardening, as so often in life, what's missing is another layer and it need not be a time-consuming one. You could add a bulb layer so that, come late winter, there will be snowdrops winking and then daffodils, tulips, alliums. You get the drift(s). Or, if you have too many perennials (though some say that is never possible), then add a shrub or two. Other garden layers include trees, perennials (short, mid-level, tall), grasses, climbers, ramblers, and so on.

If you're suffering from humdrumitis, then why not add a layer too? Again, almost any layer will do, as long as it brings you happiness. It could be something simple and daily, such as taking a walk or reading a book or playing chess. You could take up a hobby or renew your interest in a sport that hasn't been played in ages. Perhaps you can challenge yourself to make a new recipe once a week. The world is your oyster or, should we say, garden.

How to get more shimmering moments in your life

Iridescence (and wildlife), desire for

Iridescence is a magical thing, an optical phenomenon where something seems to change colour constantly. It is not seen enough in the garden, unless you happen to be blowing bubbles or have a pet peacock who likes to dance the shimmy. Perhaps this is why it feels so special when you see the iridescent wings of a dragonfly flitting around your garden. It's just one of those sights, not unlike if you see a hummingbird, that enchant and fascinate.

Fortunately, there is a very practical way to attract iridescence into your garden. The cure is a pond, any size or shape will do. It can be as small as a bucket or a puddle, or as large as a (big) pool. You might think it will be complicated, but there is no need: you will require water, of course, and a way to retain it (recycled plastic or puddled clay if it is 'in ground'). One side needs to be a gentle slope to give frogs and toads an easy way to get out. It should be in partial shade and sun. Plant it up for the seasons – try marsh marigold (*Caltha palustris*) for spring, water mint (*Mentha aquatica*) and iris for summer, and also grasses for height. You can do this in a container, using bricks to create levels for the plants as well as some outside as a sort of staircase down. Waterlilies now come in dwarf and miniature varieties, which makes everything even lovelier.

Creating a pond is the great game-changer when it comes to attracting wildlife of all kinds to your garden. An important rule, though, is no fish as they are top predators in a pond. Instead, you may attract frogs, toads, hoverflies, water beetles, water striders, candisfly larvae – and, yes, almost certainly, dragonflies. If you want to make them feel especially at home, include some upright plants, such as flowering rush (*Butomus umbellatus*) or pickerel weed (*Pontederia cordata*) for larvae to climb up and out of the water, so they can open their glittering wings for the very first time. It's a small drama but a thrilling one.

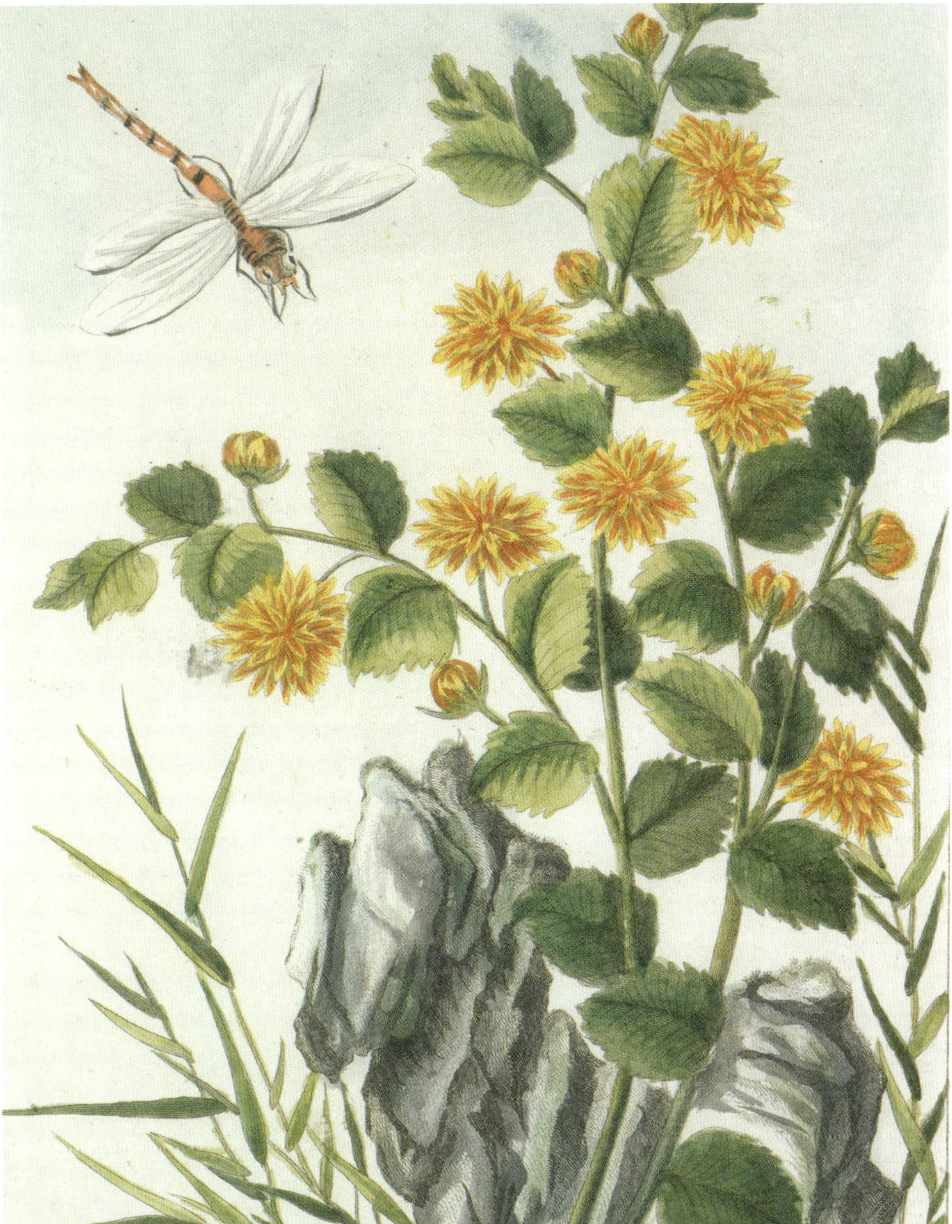

Dragonfly with *Chrysanthemum indicum* by Pierre Joseph Buchoz, from *Collection Précieuse et Enluminée Des Fleurs...*, Vol. 2, 1776.

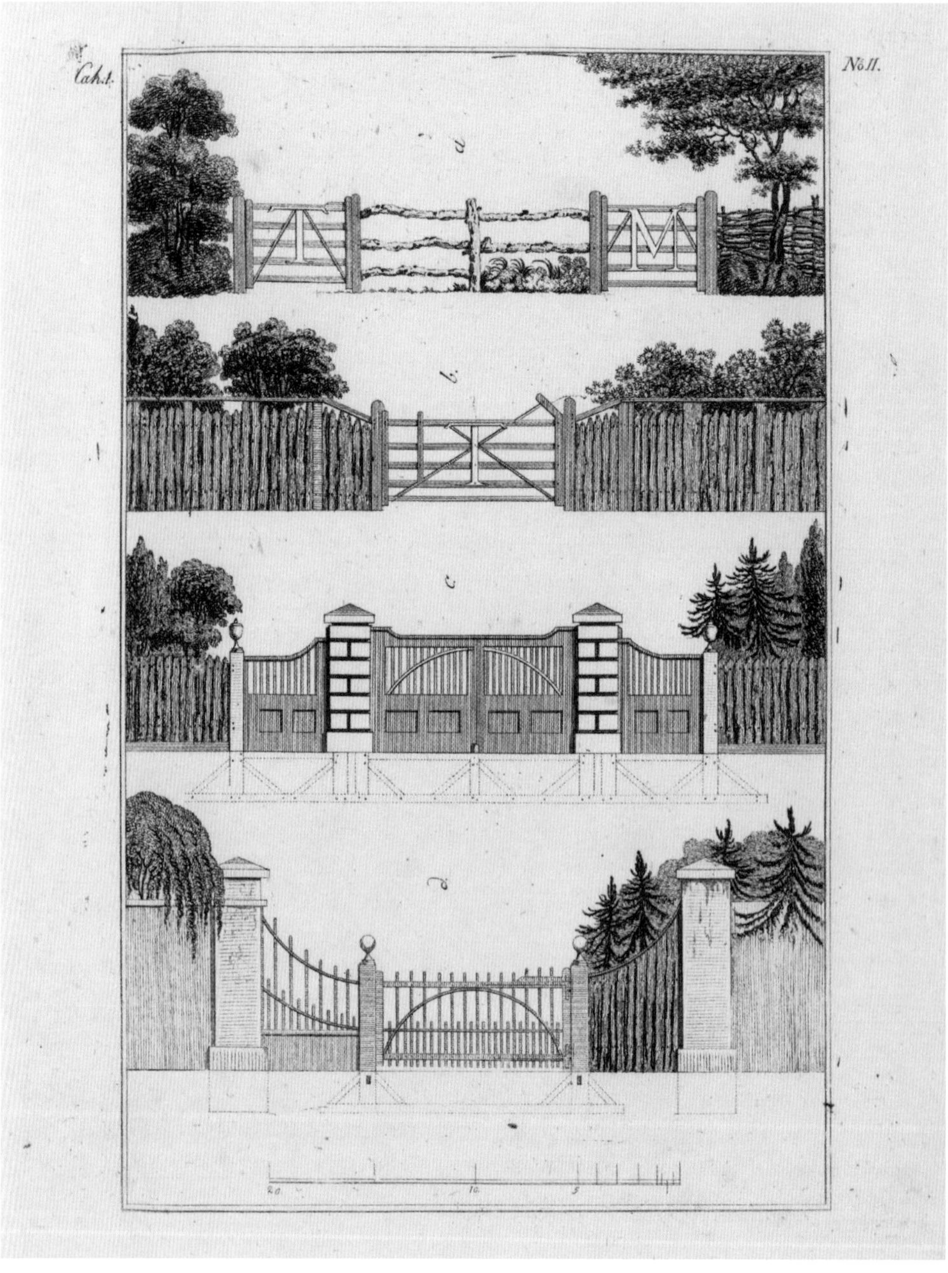

Gate designs by Johann Gottfried Grohmann, from *Ideenmagazin für Liebhaber von Gärten...*, 1797.

Every day can be a grand day to enter your own home

Make an entrance, desire to

When you enter a room, do you like it when all eyes are on you? When you go to a party, do you enter with a flourish, a hug, an exclamation? When you see a grand staircase, do you have the desire to walk down it, slowly, elegantly, stylishly? If any of these are true, then you like to make an entrance. You like a bit of drama and, perhaps, even a touch of grandeur.

Everyday life can be lacking in opportunities to make an entrance, but don't let that stop you. You can make a dramatic entrance every day, indeed several times a day, into your very own home via your garden, whatever size it is. Think symmetry. Stylish paving. Bold planting. Straight lines.

Install a (low) ironwork gate which could instantly up the formal factor. The Romans were keen on a triumphal arch, but that could seem a bit over the top these days. Instead, make a statement path to your front door and flank it with rows of lavender or catmint (*Nepeta*). Or plant yew balls and teepees with bulb underplanting. For grandeur, border the path with matching trees. If you have a tiny front garden, then go for two shrubs or, if possible, trees and make them special. Think evergreen as in bay, yew or pencil cypress, or trees with beautiful bark such as the West Himalayan birch (*Betula utilis* subsp. *jacquemontii*). If you prefer something flowerful, ornamental cherries (*Prunus*) add springtime glamour.

What a great feeling it is to walk up this front path (up-light the trees for added ooh là là) and almost be able to hear the trumpets announcing your arrival. Don't be shy when it comes to the front door either. Go for a bold colour and don't shrink away from the idea of a lion's head door knocker. It's all about drama and, well, you. And why not?

Follow your inner Capability Brown to make all things curved

Make an entrance full of surprises, desire to

When you enter a room, do you prefer to sidle in, as if you aren't making an entrance at all? At a party, do you like to arrive unannounced and then delight in surprising your host? Does the idea appeal to you of hiding behind a pillar and just – whoosh! – appearing? When faced with any space, do you often take the long way round? If so, you have the kind of spirit that would appeal to Capability Brown in the 18th century who never saw a path that he didn't want to curve.

If you happen to own an estate, then you can create an entrance the Capability Brown way with a long, meandering drive. Ideally, there will also be an undulating river, not too wide, to allow for graceful stone bridges. Along the way, there will be diverting views – of a folly, say, or a clump of trees (the skirts of which will all be trimmed to the same height). There are no fences (more surprises!) because of the ha-ha. This is how Brown, a visionary, saw things, and in his eyes all entrances were round-about and an experience in themselves.

If you don't have an estate, then you will have to downsize the plan somewhat, and possibly forgo the undulating river, but you can still create a sense of mystery and delight. An arch or low gate will signal that you have started your journey. Curve the path if possible. Indeed, curve everything. Create pocket views of planting, preferably naturalistic. Grasses, perennials. It would be great to feel as if you are flowing, not walking, to your own front door. A tree will give height and perspective but go for one or three. We don't want symmetry but surprise. Make your entrance an experience in itself.

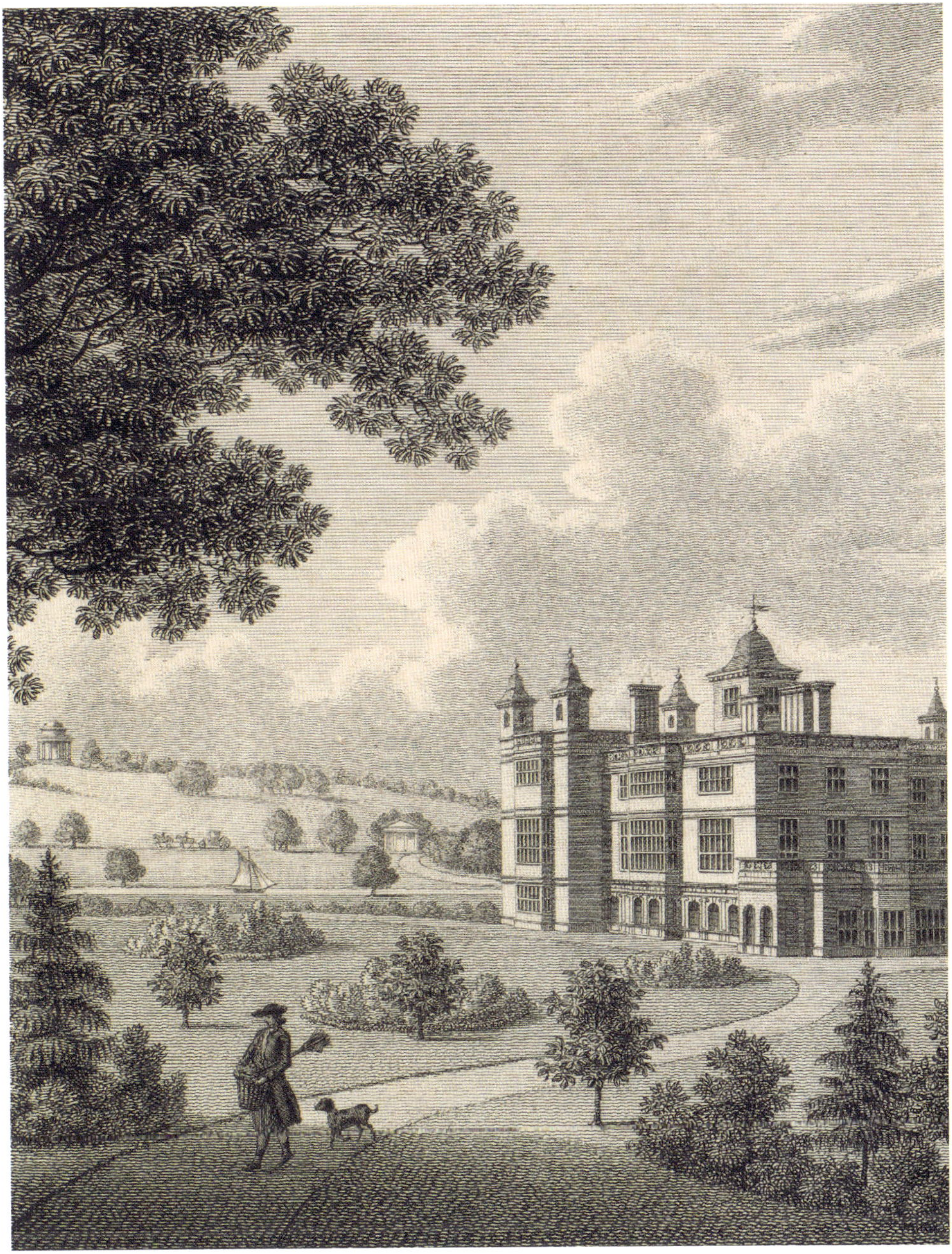

Audley End House, in Essex, with grounds designed by Capability Brown. Print by William Watts, from *The Seats of Nobility and Gentry*, c.1779.

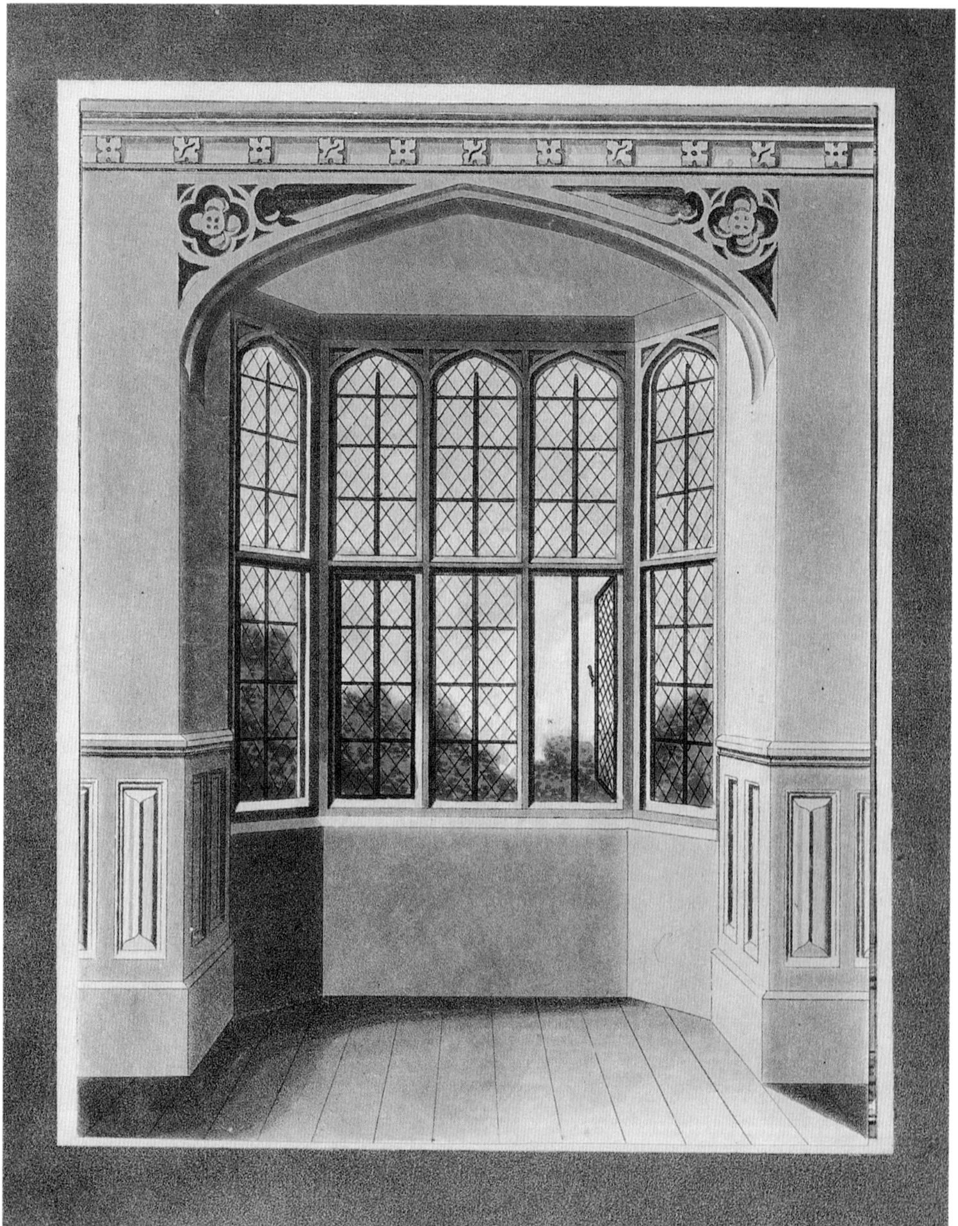

A window at Barningham Hall, Norfolk, by Humphry Repton, from *Fragments on the Theory and Practice of Landscape Gardening*, 1816.

Look out your window and be thankful if you can see green

In hospital, finding yourself

If you find yourself in hospital, for whatever reason, then it is important to remember that you don't need to be in an actual garden to garner some of its benefits. All's you really need to do is to be able to see it. We have Roger S Ulrich, a professor of architecture, to thank for this knowledge. His studies have profoundly influenced the design of health centres and hospitals around the world and improved the recoveries of countless patients.

It all goes back to Ulrich's study, published in 1984, which was conducted at an unnamed hospital in Pennsylvania in the eastern USA. The hospital was chosen for its layout: one wing had rooms that were almost identical on both sides except for the view out of the window, which was either a brown brick wall or a small stand of trees. The study was conducted over 9 years with 46 patients who were matched for age, sex, weight and general health histories. All had the same surgery (gallbladder removal) between late spring and mid-autumn when the trees were in leaf.

The results showed that patients with the tree view had significantly better recoveries with a shorter length of hospitalization, decreased use of pain medications and better moods and behaviours. Since 1984, the research into the effect of natural views on hospital recovery has widened and deepened, but the basic premise – a room with a green view makes you better faster – remains the same. It's amazing but true. Many hospitals have now created garden spaces on the inside as well as outside and have found ways to include plants, as seen through glass panels or screens, as part of the décor. It's a way to make you better, almost magically.

If you feel the need to paint your face, think woad

Be someone else, desire to

Do you wake up occasionally and think 'I feel like leading a war of independence today!' and then put on some tartan and swashbuckle around the house like you are someone who swashbuckles all the time? You may have heard of something called imposter syndrome when someone can't believe they can do the things that they actually do. Well, this swashbuckling is quite the opposite: your goal is to be an actual imposter. Others call it something more respectable – that is, acting. It's a perfectly accepted distraction from real life, though you need to pick your moments. There is no point impersonating William Wallace on a trip to Waitrose.

Your garden 'cure' is actually more an ally. It's woad, as in *Isatis tinctoria,* an ancient dyer's herb which is also quite handy in a poultice to treat wounds, helping to stop bleeding and drying them out. It was grown commercially for ages as it was, along with madder (red) and weld (yellow), and used widely to dye clothing until synthetic dyes were discovered in more recent times. In the garden, woad itself is a bit of an imposter: it has green leaves and a yellow (late spring) flower. It's only when you boil the leaves, do you start to see blue.

There is some discussion about whether William Wallace really painted his face with woad but, for theatrical purposes, it certainly made Mel Gibson look like the real deal. It's generally thought that some ancient Britons found woad face paint made them scarier. The recipe involves crushed woad leaves and a binder such as egg whites or beef fat. You have to grow the woad, of course, though you could just buy some woad pigment and mix it with a liquid binder such as whisky, which feels very Braveheart.

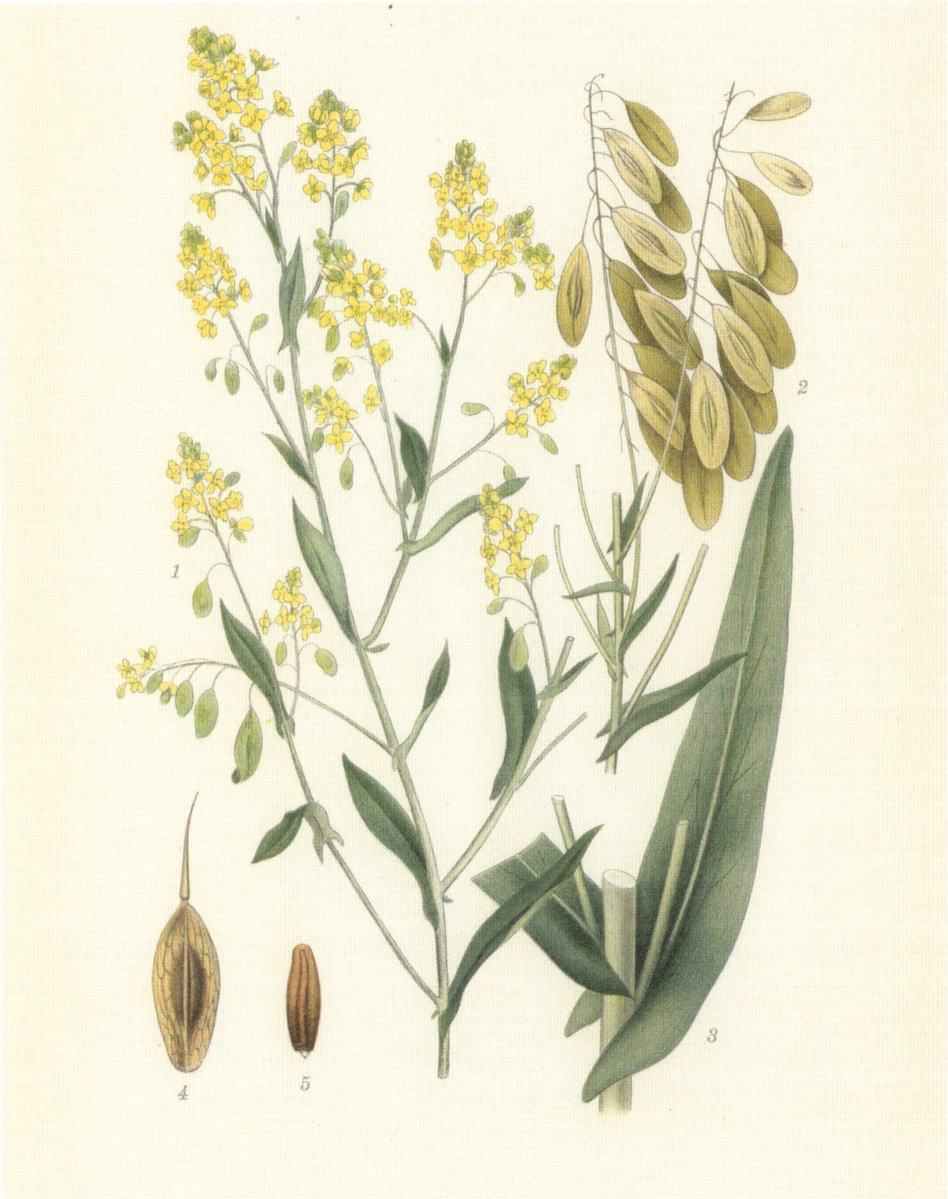

Woad (*Isatis tinctoria*) by Carl Axel Magnus Lindman, from *Bilder ur Nordens Flora*, 1922.

The job of ornamental hermit could easily make a come-back

A hermit, desire to be

There are hermits and then there are ornamental hermits. The former are the real deal, such as Paul of Thebes (227–341) who lived in a desert mountain cave in Egypt on a diet of dates and bread from the age of 16. The idea of an occupational or ornamental hermit was much more about being fashionable. What came first was the dwelling, or hermitage, a must-have feature for grand Georgian gardens. It would be a no-frills place, made of wood or stone, occasionally with actual tree roots and branches involved. The first English one was created, complete with druidic grove, by physician and antiquarian William Stukeley in Grantham, Lincolnshire, in 1727. William Kent made a grander version for George II's consort Queen Caroline in what is now Kew Gardens. It no longer stands but his sham garden folly at Stowe, in Buckinghamshire, remains, with its dilapidated turret.

Hermitages were often furnished to create the impression that they were occupied. Favourite props included a pair of spectacles, an open book, a pipe, a skull (symbol of immortality), all arranged as if the resident had just nipped out for a mystical stroll. It was only a matter of time before owners of estates decided that every hermitage needed an actual human hermit in it. 'Nothing, it was felt, could give such delight to the eye as the spectacle of an aged person, with a long grey beard and a goatish rough robe,' wrote Edith Sitwell in her 1933 book *English Eccentrics*.

Ornamental hermits fell out of fashion some time ago but that doesn't mean you can't become one. It's the ultimate WFH (working from home) job, after all. There's no reason why a garden shed can't become a hermitage. Skulls are not so easy to come by these days, but there are very good fakes. Anyway, it shouldn't be about the props really. It's about living a quiet, contemplative life, a rustic existence free from the trappings of wealth. It's about being in touch with nature and spirituality and – of course – yourself.

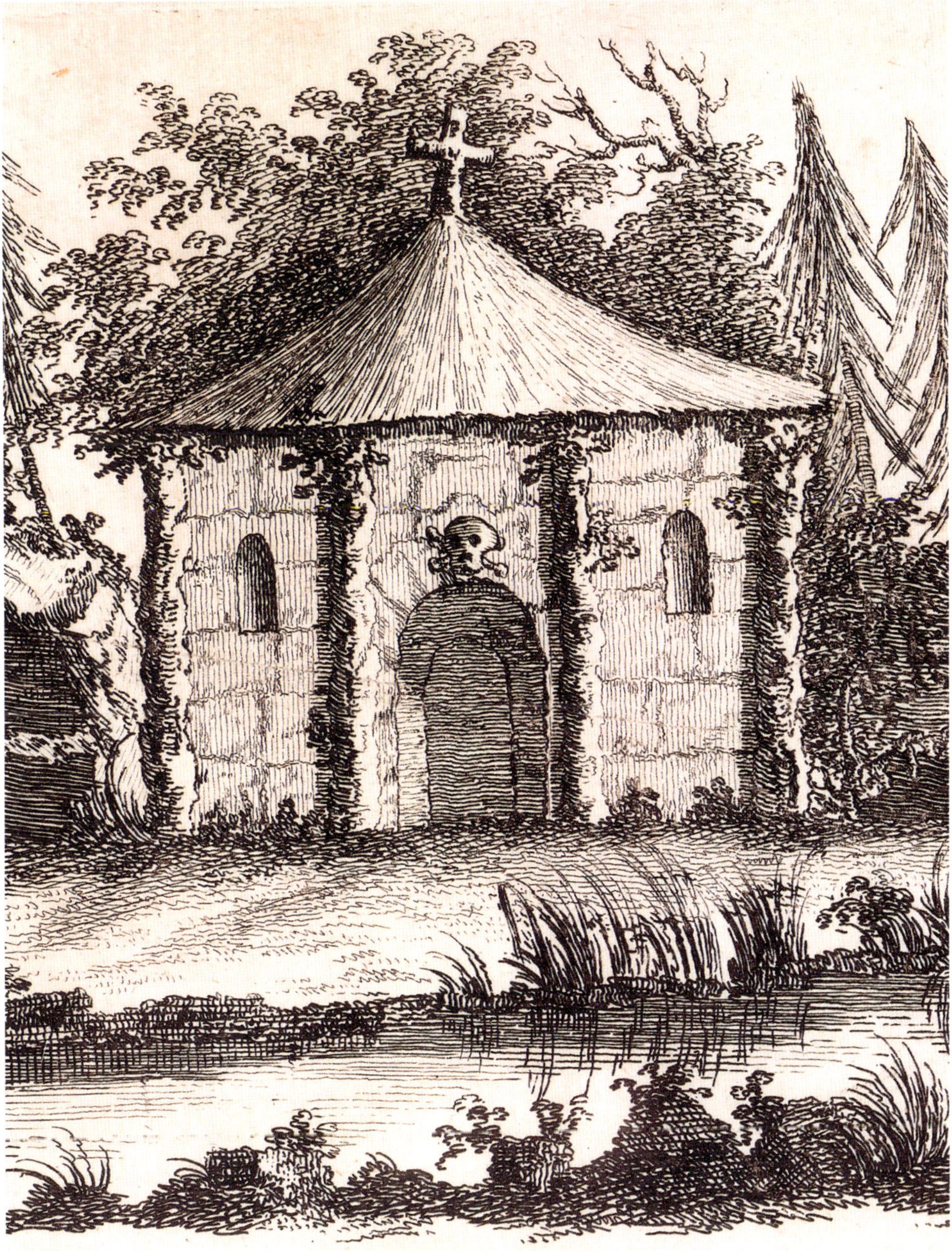

A hermit's cell by A. Thornthwaite, from
William Wrighte's *Grotesque Architecture*, 1767.

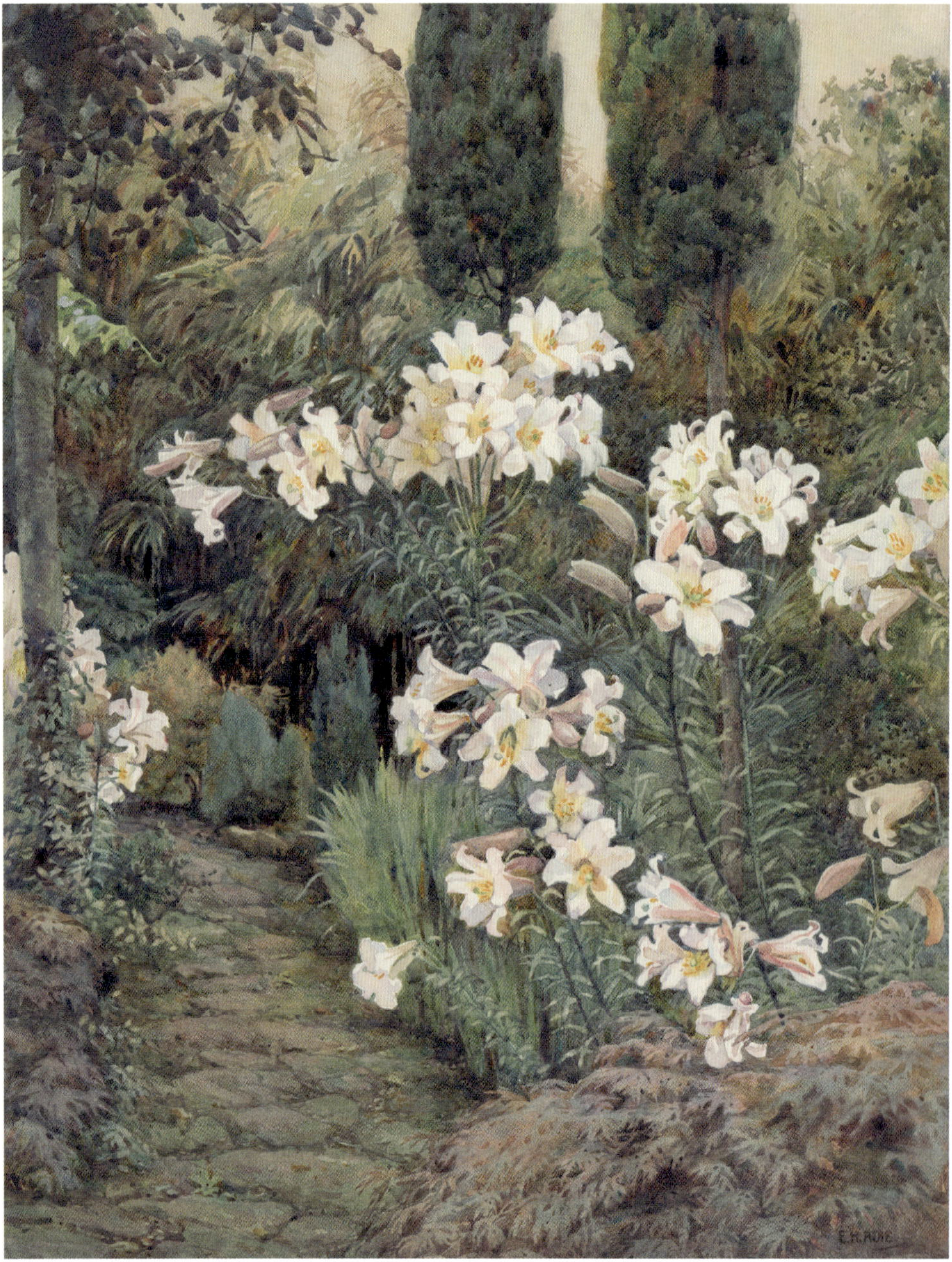

Consider the Lilies, Dyffryn, watercolour on board of *Lilium regale* by Edith Helena Adie, 1923.

Time is on your side in a garden

Grief, seeking relief from

Grief is both a robber and giver of time. It's often the 'wrong time' for grief in everyday life, with its work schedules and social requirements. Sometimes, though, for those who are grieving, there are days and nights which never seem to end. In a garden, however, time can be a shapeshifter. You can go out to the garden for a moment and stay for an hour, or longer. You set out with the idea of doing one thing, such as picking some flowers for a bouquet, but on the way see a plant that needs repotting, or watering, or deadheading. Before you know it, a considerable amount of time has passed, and you have forgotten your original purpose anyway. The ability to absorb time in this way can be of great soothing value to grief.

The process of grieving is different for everyone, but it is usually reliably unreliable. One day can be fine, the next devastating. It's a roller-coaster and it doesn't feel like anyone, and certainly not the person grieving, is in charge. The garden provides a liminal space in all sorts of ways. Here, you can be yourself, doing your own thing in your own time. There is no one to judge if tears fall into the flower bed or there are cries of pain and frustration. You can attack the ground with vehemence or just sit and sift through a little mulch. Here, you can be alone, freed from the requirements of people who want to say the right thing but usually don't, yet not lonesome. You can talk to the dead in a garden and no one else will hear.

Gardens are unique in that there is a job to fit almost all forms of grief. Sometimes you just need somewhere to sit and be (some people have a 'grief bench'), but often having an activity of some kind helps. It can be pleasing to spread mulch or create a path with wood chips, which requires endless wheelbarrow trips. Many tasks, including weeding, involve mindless repetition which can be soothing. Some tasks involve ladders and hand pruners, and erecting trellises, and require only a brief ability to focus. Then there are those days when the thing you need most is to lose yourself for the better part of a day battling to extract the roots of a tiresome and ever-spreading plant like bamboo.

Flowers for the funeral and memories in the garden

Grief, finding a way through

Many of the rituals of death involve the garden and flowers. Which ones are most often used in funerals or other ceremonies depends on the country, as well as the person. In Europe, both white lilies and roses are common choices. In Mexico, the Aztec marigold (*Tagetes erecta*) is the flower of the dead, used to decorate altars – their vibrant colour and scent is thought to guide the spirits of the dead home. Chrysanthemums, particularly white ones, are especially used in Asia. None of these are of relevance if personal preferences are involved: Queen Victoria threw the usual lilies and roses out the window when she sent a wreath of primroses to Prime Minister Benjamin Disraeli's funeral in 1881. They were his favourite flower, especially the wild ones. One especially heartfelt way to remember someone is to plant a tree/shrub/flower that can be seen from a memory bench. It can provide comfort, whatever the season.

Getting down to earth can provide comfort

Grief, digging in to let go of

There is something obviously grounding about a garden because it (usually) involves quite a lot of soil. Some people say that, after a trauma or a deep loss, what they want to do is to get their hands in the soil. They get rid of the garden gloves and dig in, with their fingernails. They go barefoot, experiencing the earth and grass with their feet, a process that can involve soles and souls. There is something else about soil that helps those who are grieving. Soil contains microbes, including *Mycobacterium vaccae*, which when inhaled or touched have been found in multiple studies to make us feel better. It's all linked to the hormone serotonin, which can stabilize moods and boost positive feelings. When we absorb *Mycobacterium vaccae*, through contact with soil, it activates a small group of neurons that contain serotonin. It works as a natural antidepressant and, for the grieving, is always a plus.

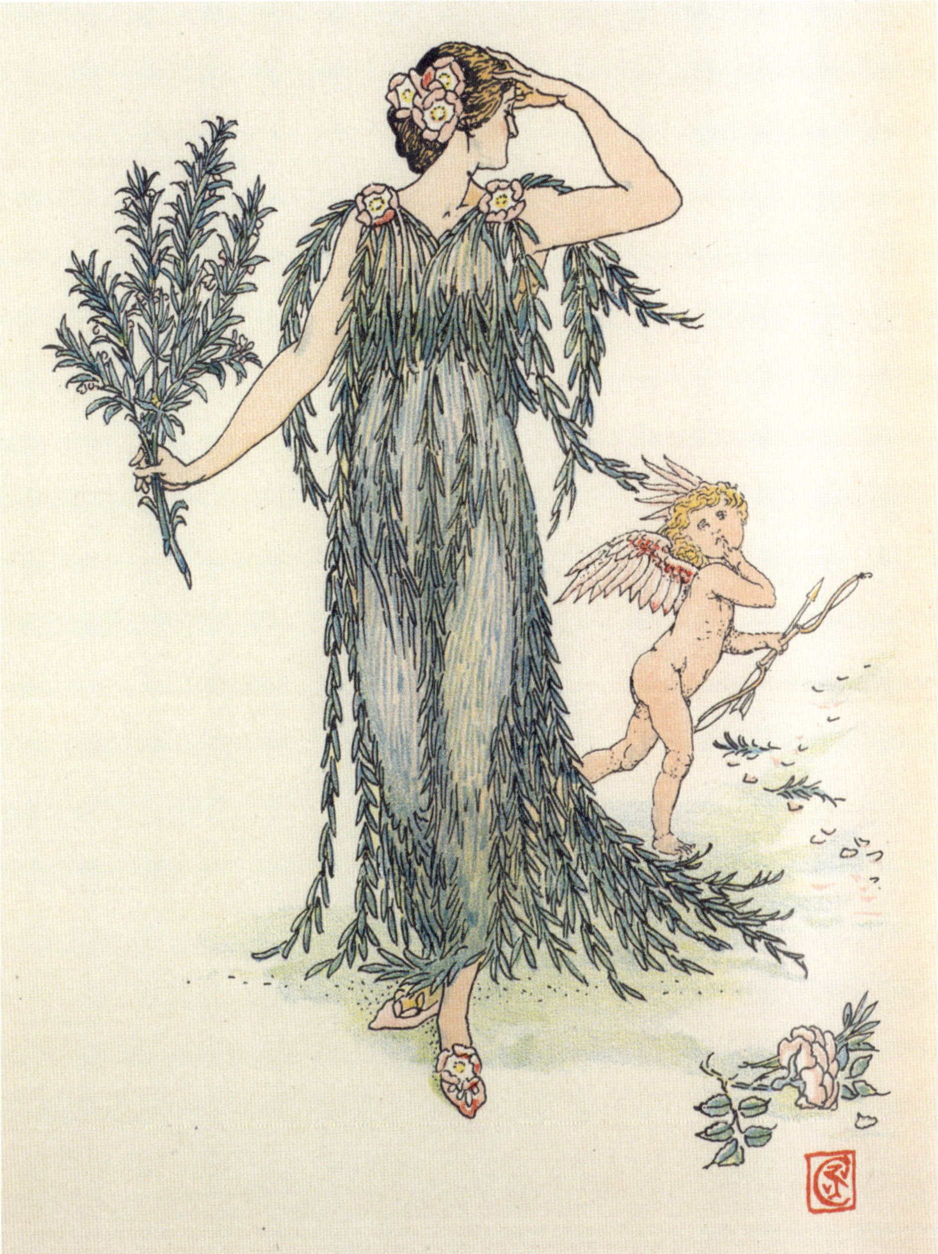

Ophelia's lament: 'There's rosemary, that's for remembrance'. Walter Crane illustrates *Hamlet* in *Flowers from Shakespeare's Garden*, 1906.

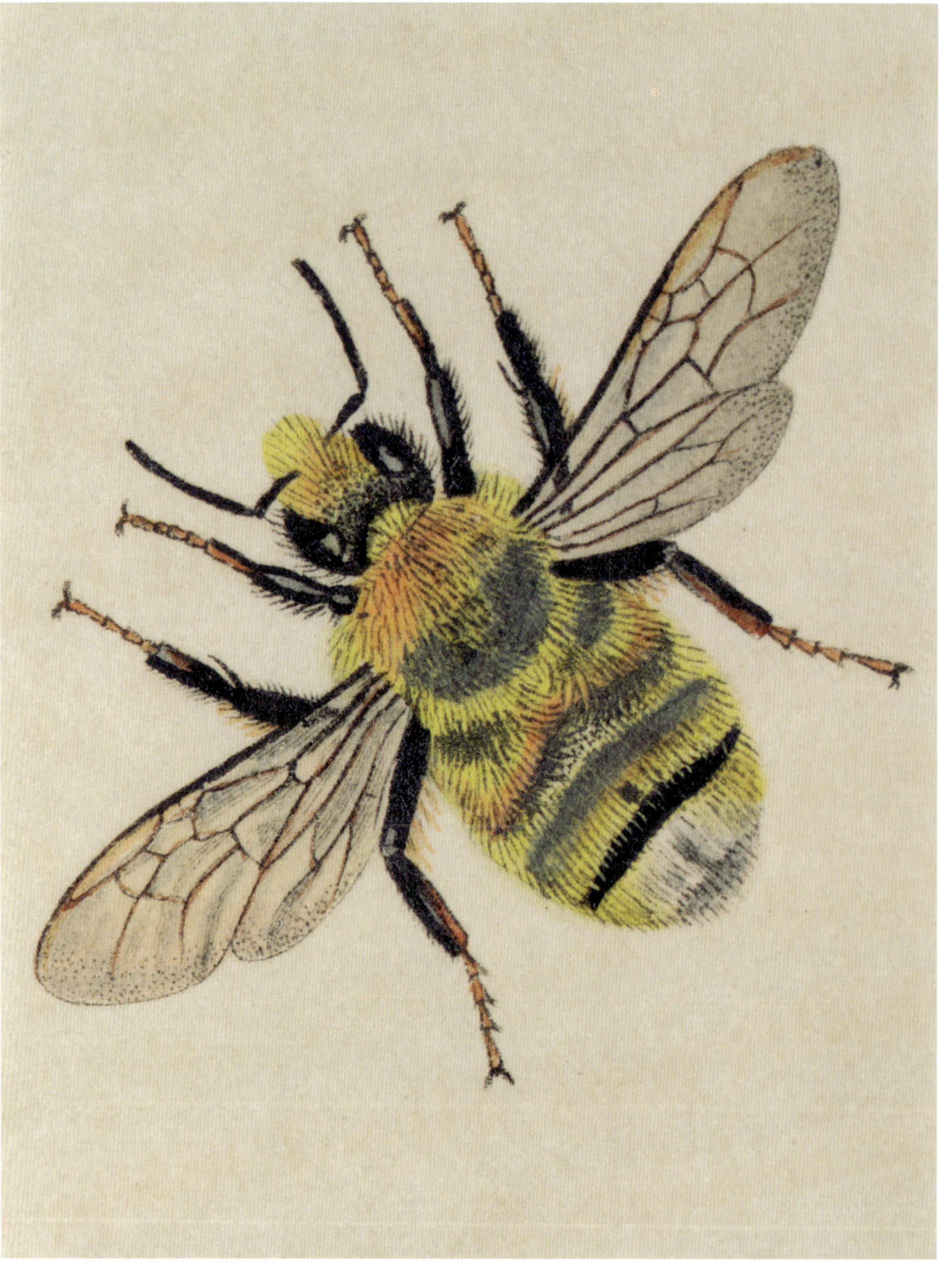

Tree bumblebee (*Bombus hypnorum*) by John Curtis, from *British Entomology...*, Vol. 6, 1823–40.

A bee can provide us with a completely different outlook

A new perspective, finding

At times it is difficult to remember that everyone sees things differently. Indeed, it is a core principle of mindfulness to try and see things from another perspective. The idea being that if we change our perspective, we can sometimes change our minds. It can lift the spirit and enlarge our world view. The garden provides a particularly dramatic example of this by helping us to try and see the world through a bee's eyes.

What we see when we look at bees is not what bees see looking back at us. For starters, they have near panoramic vision from their two large compound eyes which are made up of thousands of tubes called ommatidia. Their bee brains merge all these images into a single mosaic-type scene, but it lacks detail and will be blurred. From our perspective, we would call bees short-sighted. They also have an adaption, which when flying quickly switches their vision to black and white, thus freeing up their brains from having to process so many images. (Bees also have three smaller eyes on top of their heads that act as a sort of GPS and help with balance.)

We see colours from red to violet, but bees have a different colour spectrum which includes ultra-violet light with shorter wavelengths. Some flowers that may look plain to us will look exciting to a bee, with intricate UV spots and stripes. These patterns are often nectar guides. Bees also can't see red, which appears black or dark to them. They do see something called 'bee-purple' which is a mix of UV and yellow light. To see the world through a bee's eyes is to see something in a radically different – and beautiful – way.

Does the feeling go both ways? Ask the Fibonacci sequence

Being in love, anxious about

There are possibly more direct ways to find out if someone loves you (or not), but daisy divination has the immense plus of not requiring direct communication. Why pick up the phone or (gasp) ask directly when you can instead sit in a picturesque meadow, plucking at the petals of the ox-eye daisy (*Leucanthemum vulgare*)? We have probably been plucking daisies and chanting 'He loves me/he loves me not' since time (or flowers) began, but it was the French who gave the whole game a bit of extra ooh là là.

First rule, any daisy will do, though they don't have petals per say but multiple clusters of very small flowers called florets. In French, the game is called *effeuiller la marguerite* (plucking the daisy) and the sequence of questions is far more nuanced than the simple yes/no option. There is a range of five love stages, starting (first petal) with *'Il/elle m'aime un peu'* and moving on via two, three, four petals to *'beaucoup, passionnément, à la folie'*. Finally, there's the brutal final fifth option of *'pas du tout!'*

The good news, provided by scientists and not divination, is that it is uncommon to end with 'not at all'. This is because of the number sequence called the Fibonacci sequence which comprises the numbers 1, 1, 2, 3, 5, 8, 13, 21, 34, 55, and so on (you add the two previous numbers to get the next). This sequence rules in many flowers, including daisies, and means that most daisies will have an odd number of petals (he loves me). If you're playing the more complicated French version, then you're still in luck as you're even more unlikely to end up on 5, 10, 15, 20. Most daisies have fewer than 55 florets. Phew. I guess s/he loves you, in some way or another.

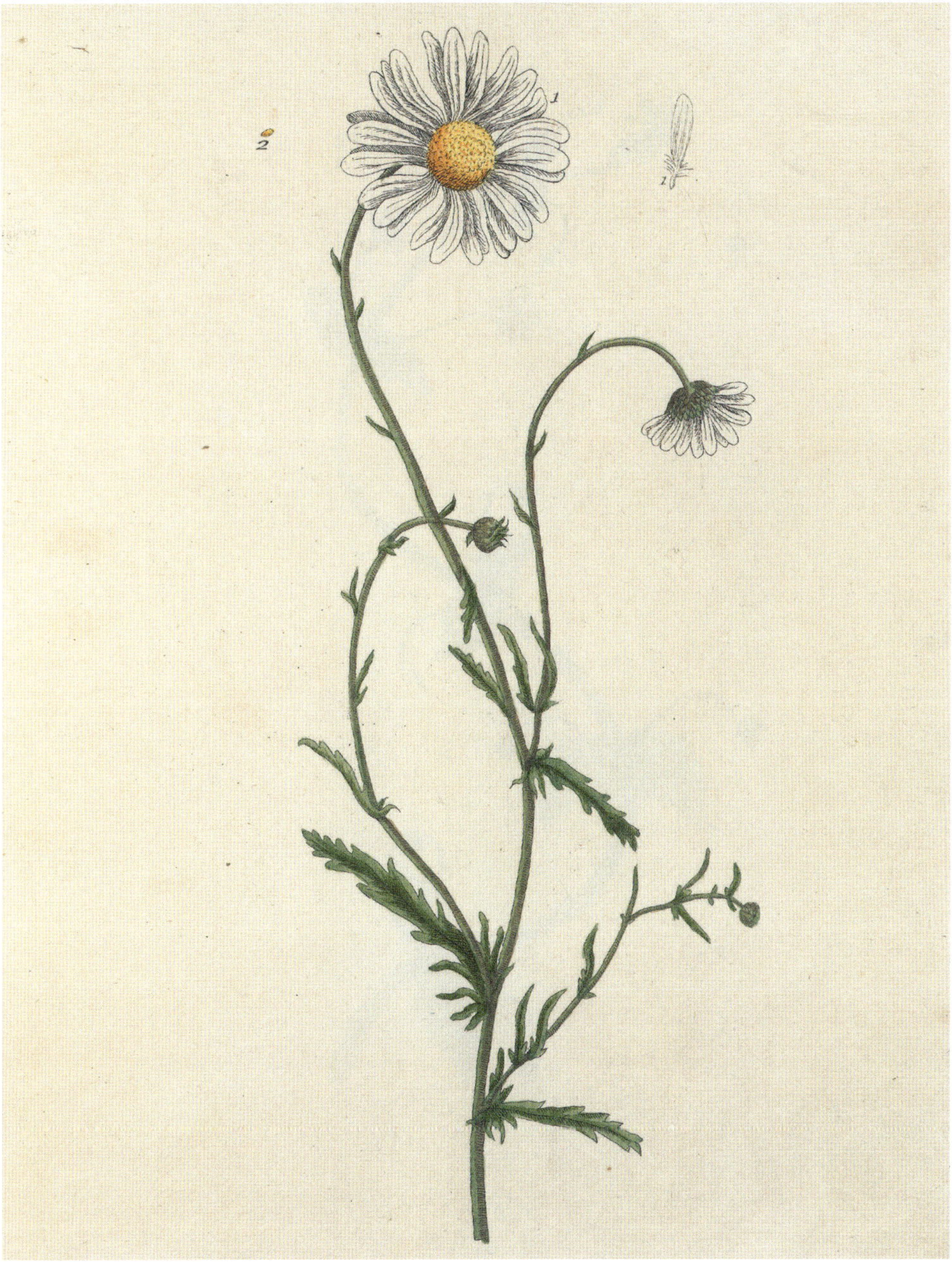

Ox-eye daisy (*Leucanthemum vulgare*) by Elizabeth Blackwell, from *A Curious Herbal*, Vol. 1, 1739.

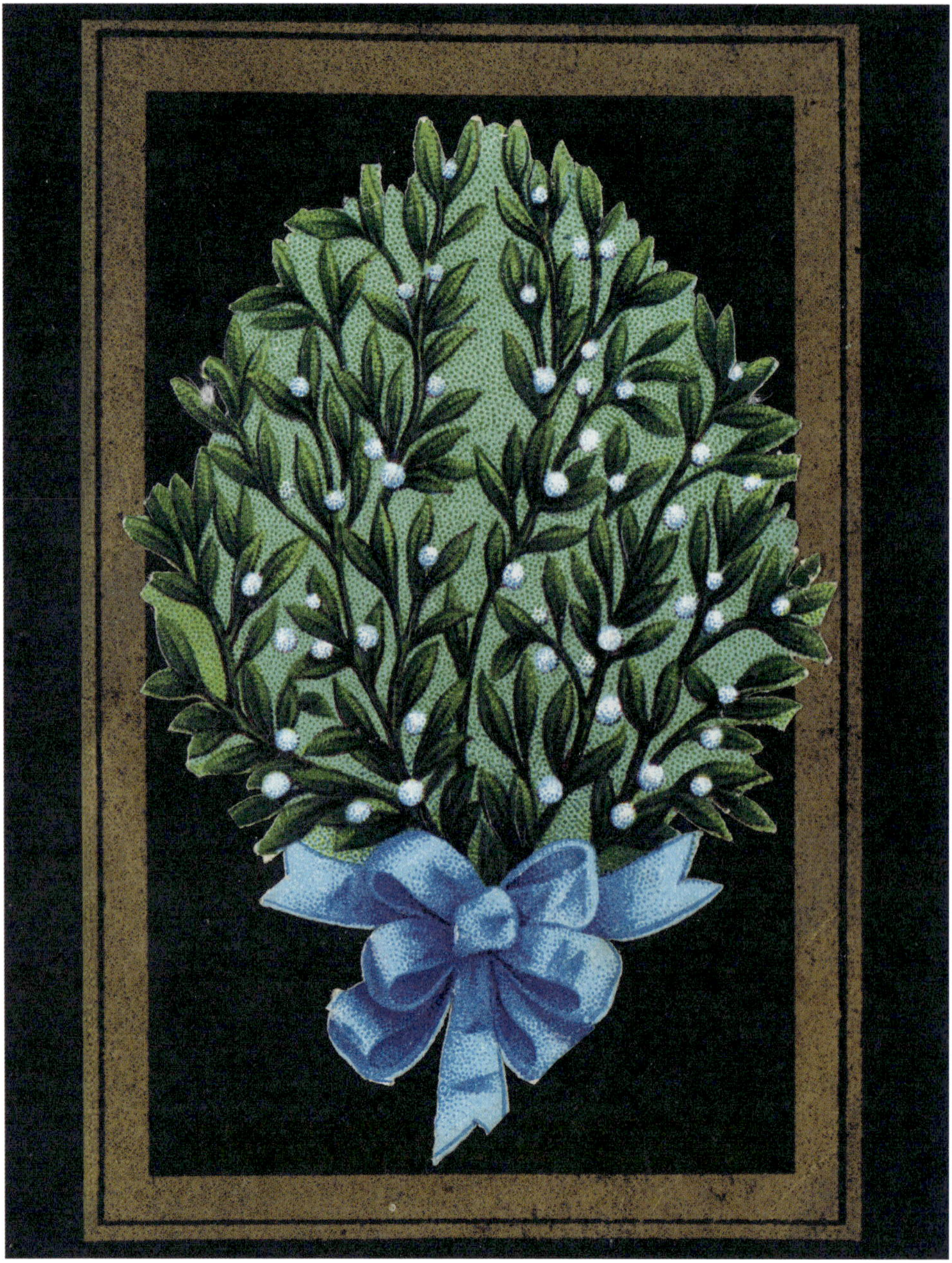

Victorian Christmas card with a bunch of mistletoe (*Viscum album*). Artist unknown.

Here's an excuse to simmer down and pucker up

Kissing, desire for

On the face of it, mistletoe (*Viscum album*) isn't the most obvious romantic choice. It's a poisonous parasitic plant that lives in trees but, then, its otherworldly factor may be the reason behind its allure. Mistletoe has no roots and, instead, taps into what amounts to the veins of its host tree (lime, hawthorn, apple and others). It uses the tree's water and nutrients but does its own photosynthesis using its bright green leaves, which means it's only a partial or hemi-parasite. The female has waxy, white berries spread by birds and especially the mistle thrush.

Mistletoe has been seen as something special for thousands of years, valued by the Greeks and Romans, the Celts and particularly the Druids. Heroes in Greek mythology needed mistletoe (the 'golden bough') to gain passage to the Underworld. The Druids saw it as a sacred plant, especially if it was found growing in an oak tree, as it kept its magical green in winter and (they thought) was infused with the tree's life force. They associated it with luck and fertility.

It's not clear how all that evolved into the custom, which became popular in Victorian times, of hanging a sprig from the ceiling, where young men and women would, if they found themselves under it, have a kiss. Custom had it that it was bad luck for a woman to refuse. The idea is said to have begun as a farmhouse tradition, or a practice among servants in larger houses, and was spread in the writings of the likes of Charles Dickens and Washington Irving. Soon, everyone was doing it. Apparently, there are rules. You must pluck a berry for every kiss given, though, remember, they aren't to be eaten because they are poisonous.

There's one plant in particular that is all about a love lost

Heartbreak, getting over

It is only human to have our hearts broken once or twice (and sometimes more) in a lifetime. There is a small industry involved in advising us how to mend a broken heart – forget him/her, find another, go for a run, go on a trip, eat ice cream, drink champagne, find a new hobby – but there is no known cure. Sometimes it's best to do nothing and to remember that a broken heart is the price we pay for love. Would you rather not love? (Wait, don't answer that.)

It may help to think of a broken heart as something of which to be proud – a badge of sorts – and there is one plant that, in the garden, will remind you that you have been there, done that, and have weathered the storm (or will soon). It is *Lamprocapnos spectabilis,* previously *Dicentra*, which is commonly known as 'Bleeding Heart'. It's native to northeast China and Korea and has been in Europe since Victorian times. In Asia, it is viewed as a good luck sort of plant, but in the West, it is a heartbreaker, epitomized as such by its long racemes of dangling teardrop flowers, of pink and red, drooping gracefully and (or so it can seem) sadly. In Germany, it is known as *Tranende Herzen* or 'Tearing Heart'. It likes shade, which fits in well with heartbreak in general, and is an early spring perennial, popping up when other flowers are still sleeping, its pendulous flowers reminding us of what has been.

'Would you rather not love? (Wait, don't answer that.)'

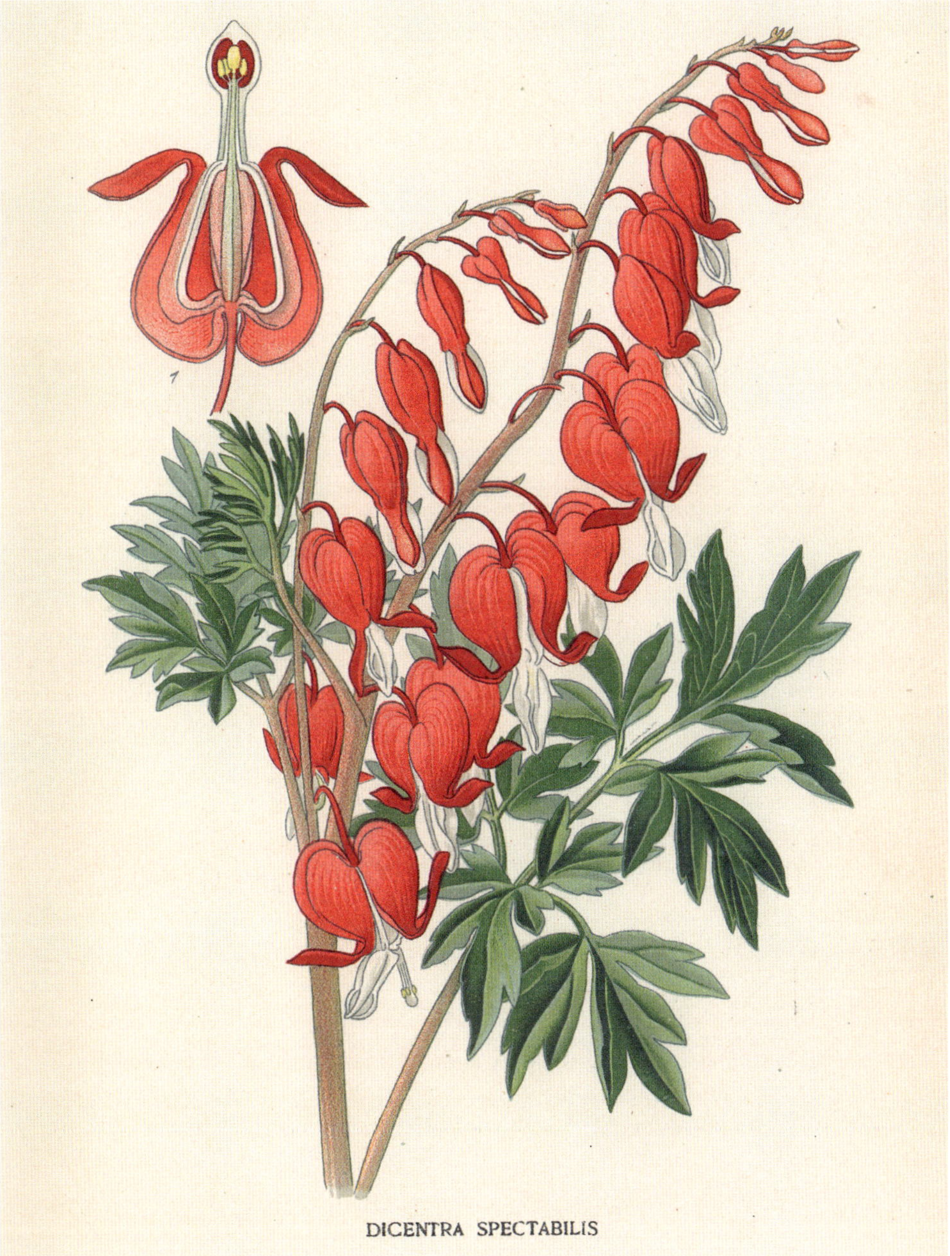

Bleeding Heart (*Lamprocapnos spectabilis*) by Edward Step,
from *Favourite Flowers of Garden and Greenhouse*, 1896–1897.

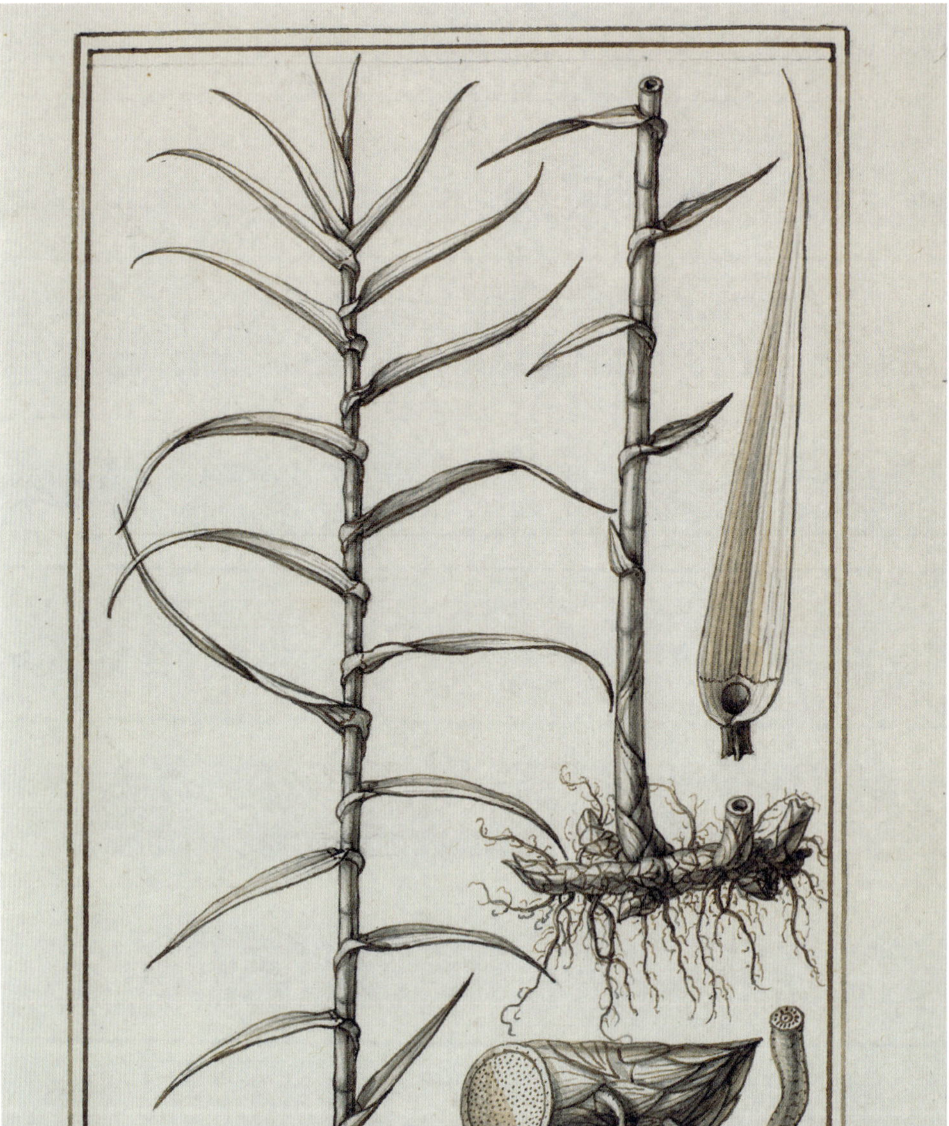

Giant reed (*Arundo donax*), pen and ink on paper by Claude Aubriet, *c*.1700.

The giant cane can lull you with its melodic purpose

Music, finding solace in

When you see a large clump of *Arundo donax*, with its tall canes swaying in the wind, the first thing that pops into your head is probably not Mozart's Serenade No. 10 (or *Gran Partita*), but perhaps it should be. This is one of the most famous works written for a wind ensemble, which, in this case, includes two oboes, two bassoons, two clarinets and two alto/tenor clarinets. All these instruments use either single or double reeds in their mouthpieces which, when blown on, vibrate and create the sound waves for pieces by Mozart or, indeed, all woodwind composers.

All natural reeds for instruments come from the *Arundo donax* or giant cane. The plant is not, it must be said, popular with everyone. It is sometimes confused with bamboo and grows up to 5m (16ft) high, with large, arching, strap-shaped leaves. It can form huge colonies that cover hundreds of acres and is considered to be invasive in some countries. It is a multi-tasker, being used to arrest soil erosion on canals and sometimes to create a windbreak. It can also be used to make brooms, pipestems, roofing and walking sticks, and in basket-weaving. But the most sublime use, by far, is to make the single and double reeds that are used in saxophones, clarinets and other woodwinds (as well as bagpipes) around the world. There are various *Arundo donax* plantations for reeds in Europe, the US, Australia and China. Maestro, please!

Lavender has the wow factor – and so much else

Superblooms, desire to find

The horticultural phenomenon known as a wild superbloom is a thrilling experience around the world. Part of its allure is its unpredictability. The hills and mountains of California may or may not turn orange for as far as the eye can see, a result of millions of *Eschscholzia californica*, or California poppies, bursting into bloom. Superblooms tend to take place in desert locations and depend on several factors which include gentle (not tumultuous) autumn rainfall, spring warmth and a lack of drying winds. If conditions are right, the results are stunning, but this can be something that happens once in 15 years. When it does occur, people arrive in droves, by helicopter even, to stand and even lie among the flowers, trampling the very thing they came to admire. It can be, as it is termed, a poppy apocalypse.

The likes of China and Japan don't leave it to chance, though: they create agricultural superblooms or 'flower seas' by growing plants of one colour, such as 'baby blue eyes' (*Nemophila*) or yellow canola or oilseed rape (*Brassica napus* subsp. *oleifera*), in huge swathes. It's all for tourists and, of course, is much more predictable (and profitable) than the wild version. In Europe, and some other places, there is an equivalent in the form of fields of tulips or sunflowers, which attract crowds but are also grown for horticultural purposes.

The star of the devised superbloom, however, is the lavender farm where vast fields of purple can extend all the way to the horizon. Lavender has the 'wow' factor as well as a 2,500-year-old history of cultivation, being brought to Britain by the Romans and used by the Egyptians for mummification. When Tutankhamun's tomb was opened, there was still a tinge of lavender in the air. Walking among fields of lavender – or even a pathway flanked by it – is a surround-smell experience. Lavender has a fresh but floral, and slightly sweet, scent that is widely seen as calming. It's beautiful – and hard-working. It is used in skincare, perfumes, home sprays, potpourri and cooking, as well as being a mainstay in the garden. Social media 'influencers' love it, as do the bees, giving lavender that superbloom buzz.

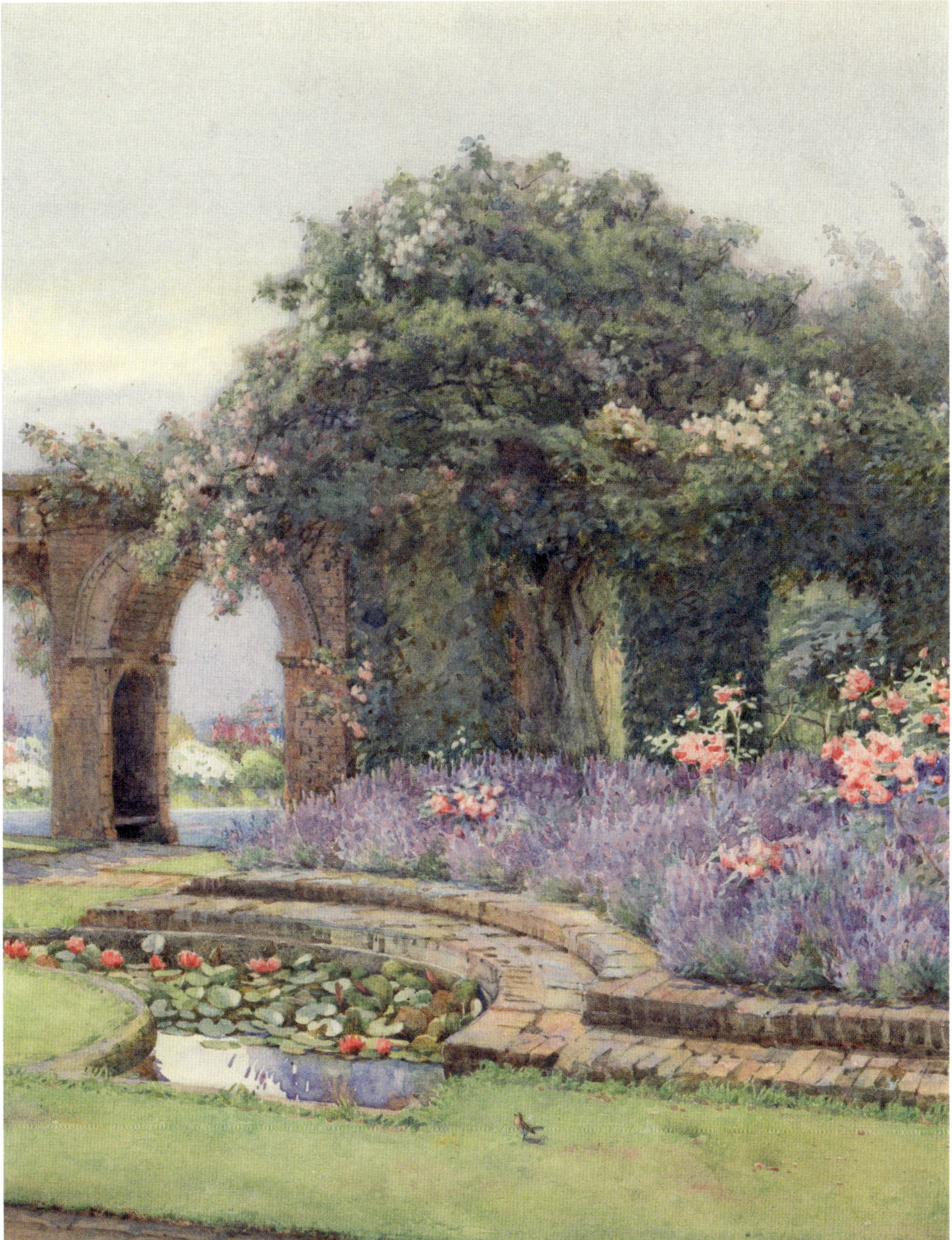

Lavender Garden, Dyffryn, watercolour on board
by Edith Helena Adie, 1923.

The answer to almost every question can be found here

Existential angst, feelings of

What is the answer to life, the universe and everything? This is the question that bedevilled the likes of Sartre and Kafka. Thankfully, Douglas Adams in *The Hitchhiker's Guide to the Galaxy* provided us with an easy-to-understand answer, as in the number 42, but it has become increasingly obvious that this answer may be incomplete. It's not clear how Sartre missed this, but the answer to almost every existential question can be found in the garden, usually behind the shed, in a bin with wooden slats and no bottom. It's the compost heap.

All of life is here. Eggshells. Cardboard. Grass clippings. Leaves. Bits of vegetable, fruit and veg that's gone way past the point of eating. Peelings. Prunings. Straw. Shredded paper. Twigs. Even your own hair. The 'green' waste is rich in nitrogen. The 'brown' stuff is rich in carbon. There are insects and, for some, the odd mouse. You just add air (turning with a fork) and water (usually rain). These are all free. Some people (mostly men) think it's great to pee on it as it will break down faster. Others just use their forks more. Pee is also free, as is everything to do with compost. You don't even really need a bin as a heap works just as well.

A well-proportioned compost heap is a beautiful thing: with layers of green and brown waste that, as it starts to break down, become increasingly intermixed and mingled. It can take six months or longer to achieve the final result, which is dark brown and rich soil. This is called 'black gold' and it's everything that it should be. It smells like the earth itself. It feels crumbly. It will provide nutrients and a home for seeds and plants to sprout and flourish. It can be used as mulch and will help the soil retain water. In a world that seems to be constantly changing, your own homemade compost will not let you down. There are a variety of ways to make compost, including something called 'hot composting' which is, literally, steamy and, well, some think is just a little bit sexy. This is the stuff of life. And it's free.

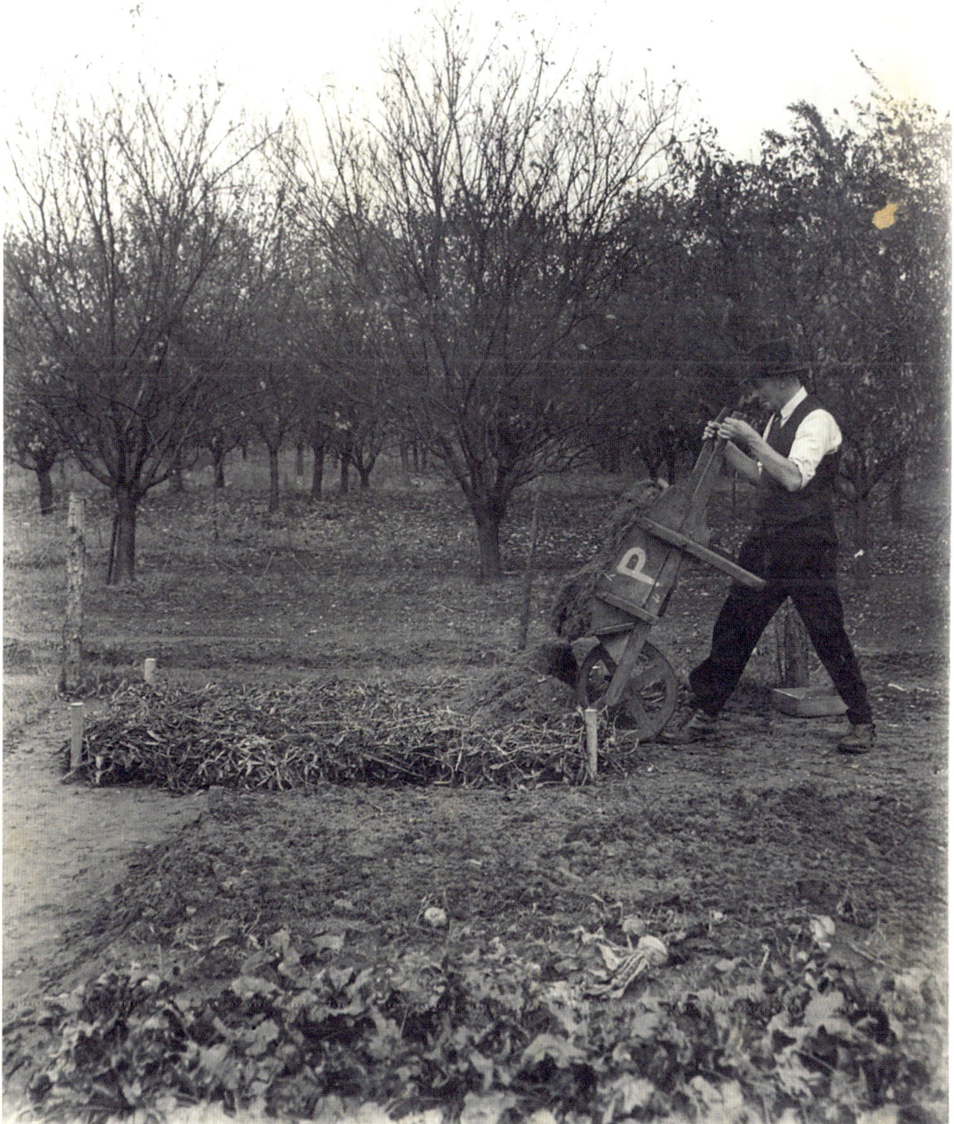

Man adding material to a compost heap, photographed by Norman Kenneth Gould or James Wilson for a 'Dig for Victory' campaign board, *c*.1943.

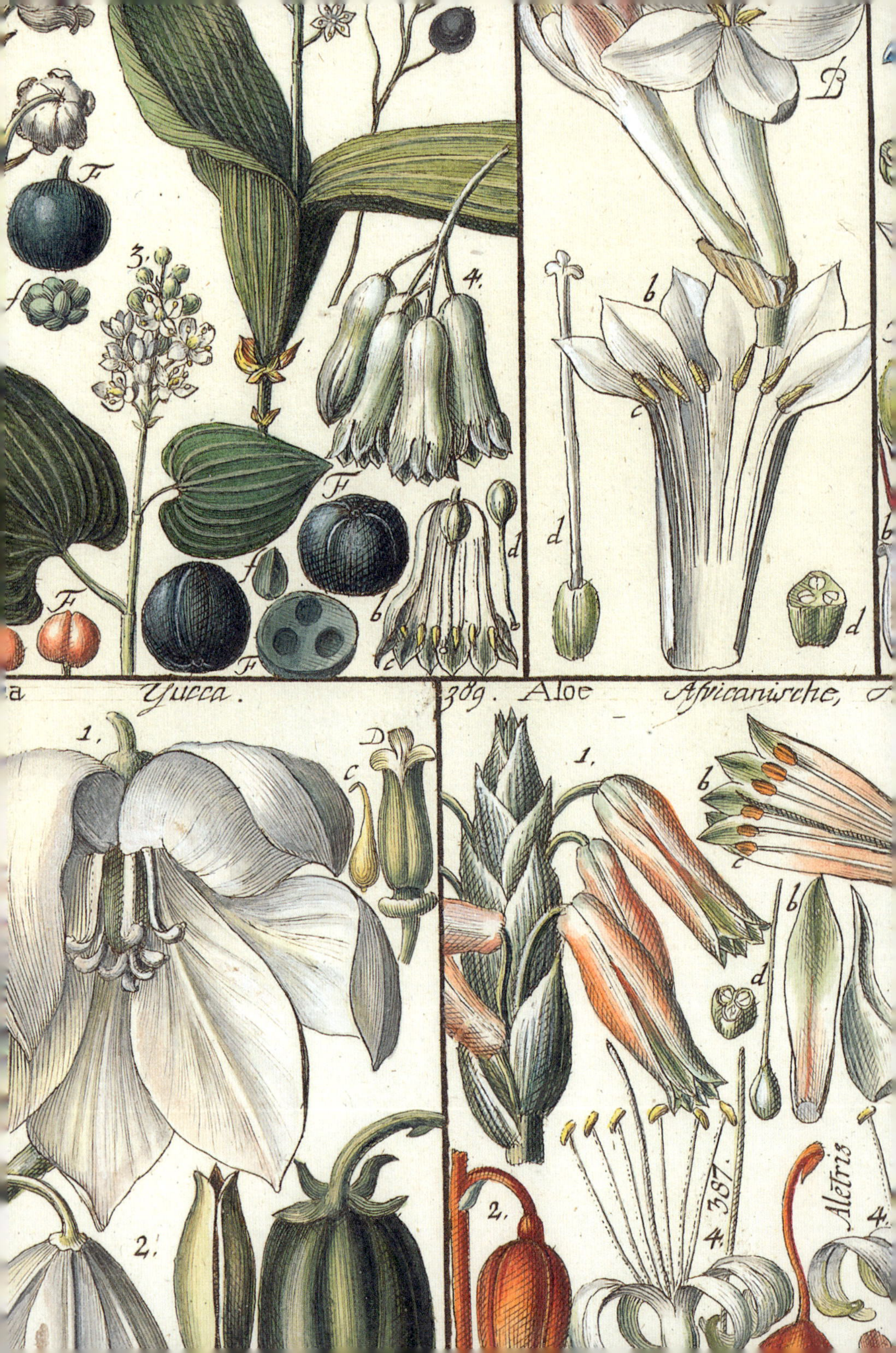
Yucca.
389. Aloe
Africanische,
387.
Aletris

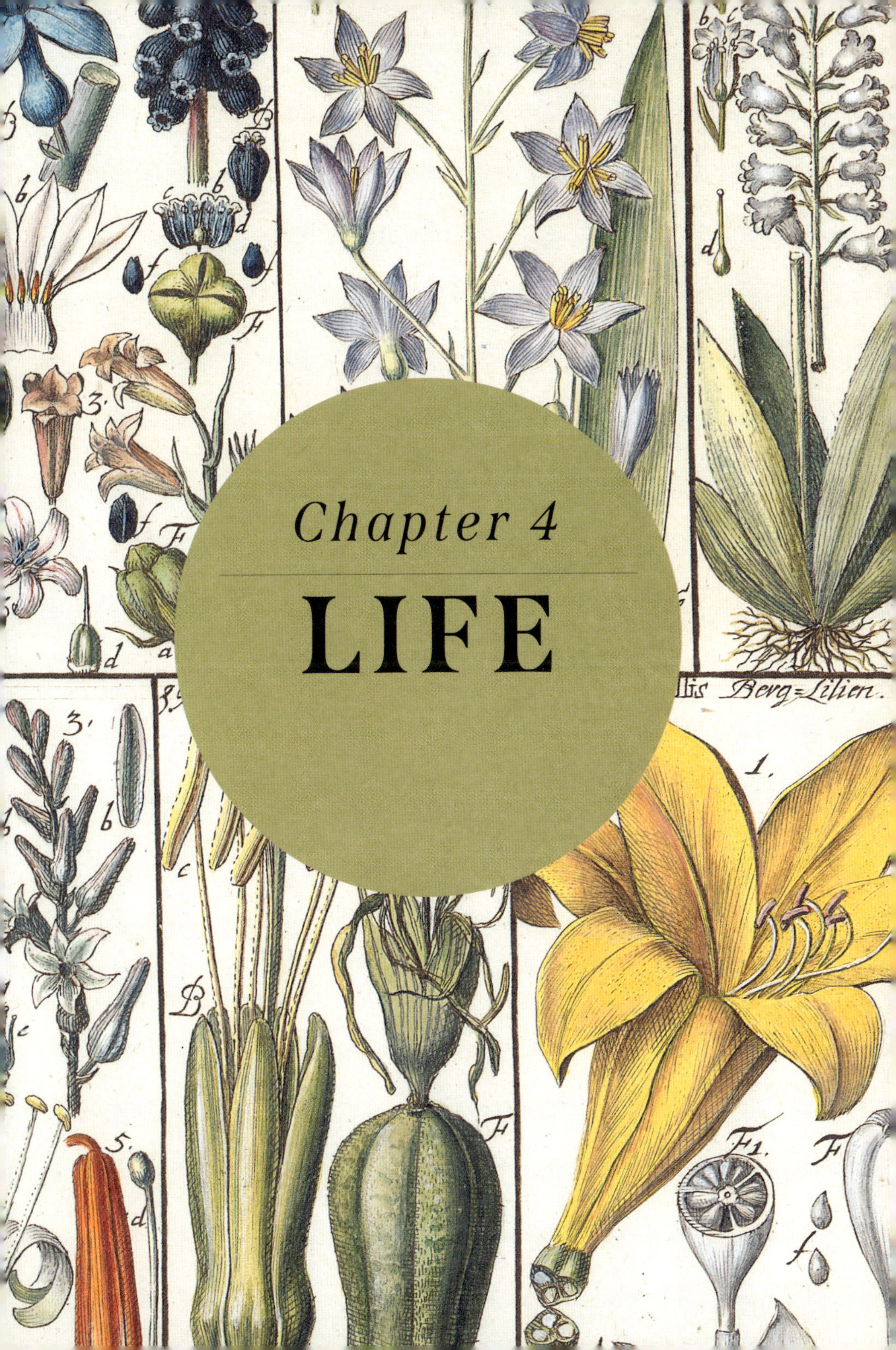

Chapter 4

LIFE

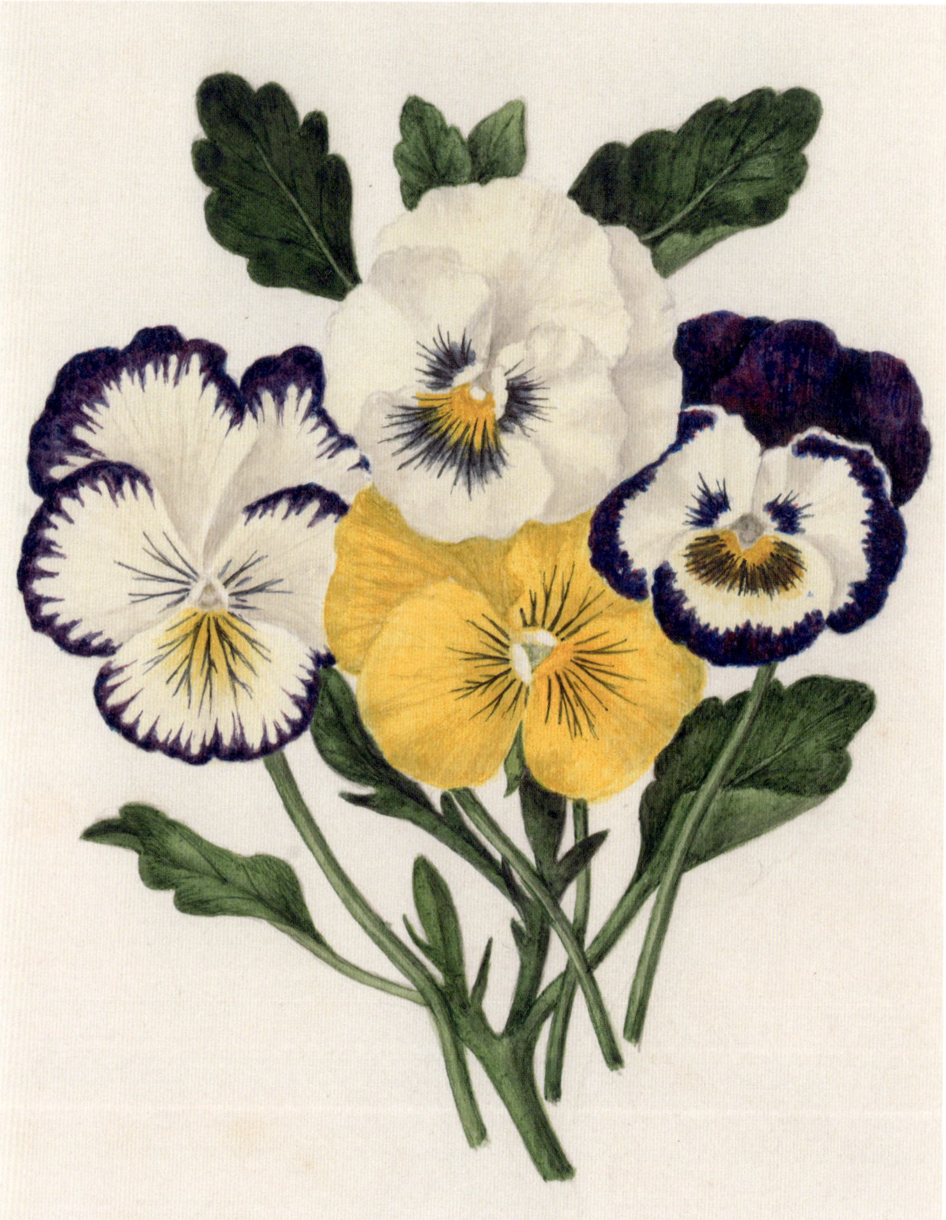

Pansies (*Viola*), watercolour on paper
by Caroline Maria Applebee, 1842.

Grow your own adorable persona

Approachable CEO, how to be an

If you are a Chief Operating Officer of anything larger than your own grocery list, then you will automatically be seen as scary. The larger the company, the scarier you will become, instantly, without doing anything. Some CEOs think this is great (see *Scary CEO, How to Be A*, page 168), but others don't like it when people look terrified. Instead, you want to be loved.

There are a variety of garden cures for this, but all involve choosing a plant that is seen as intrinsically friendly. You could develop a passion for pansies, for instance, and pair that with a love of arranging them in interesting vases. Another key factor in deciding which plant to become passionate about is that it is imperative you spread the news of your passion. So, in the pansy scenario, that would involve bringing pansy arrangements to your office and placing them in strategically obvious positions. Anyone who comes in will have to say: 'Oh, that is so pretty...' At which point, you say: 'I love pansies and, at home, I have 38 types...' (P.S. Always good to be specific because that's the kind of thing that passionate people say.)

It's imperative to seek out, and be genuinely interested in, your adorable flower subject. When it comes to pansies there's much to discover about its wild ancestor, *Viola tricolor,* which is also known by names such as 'come and cuddle me' and 'heart's ease'. The name pansy comes from the French *pensée*, meaning 'thought'. Pansies are mentioned in Shakespeare (this is a huge boon for CEOs aspiring to be loved). Feel free to quote Will S, by the way, in *Hamlet* where Ophelia says: 'And there is pansies, that's for thought'. The flowers are edible and look great scattered on cakes, though for any CEO, loved or not, bringing in a pansy-strewn cake may be going too far.

If you can't stand pansies, then pick another 'friendly' plant. Avoid all things poisonous, spiky, smelly, sticky, stingy. Also anything very large or glamorous. No one wants a CEO with a passion for gladioli. Remember that.

You want to be feared (but in a good way)

Scary CEO, how to be a

It's not something most people would admit, but there are many CEOs out there who don't mind being seen as scary. They want to be viewed as powerful to the point of formidable, but there is an issue with that: they have to attend endless meetings and functions at which they are in desperate need of a conversation topic. Thankfully, there is a garden cure for this. The garden, as we all know, provides cures of all kinds. It is not only for the kind and courteous but also for the feared and fascinating.

If you are a happily scary CEO, you need a plant passion and it's important that your plant passion be somewhat unusual. No one will be in the least fearful of someone who spends their free time obsessing over the stripes in their lawn. Make a list (or order someone else to) of plants that are charismatic and a little bit dangerous. Avoid anything actually poisonous. Developing an obsession with plants that can kill people (see *Agatha Christie, Too Much*, page 201) is something most employees would find creepy.

It's important to avoid anything that terrifies, but spiky is good. Indeed, the yucca is the perfect plant passion for the scary CEO. Yuccas are dramatic and bold, adding form and structure to any space. They range from the small and shrubby to trees such as the fascinating Joshua tree (*Yucca brevifolia*), which looks as if it has escaped from a children's storybook. Many have creamy white flower spikes that no one would call small. They are also a plant of the future, as they are xerophytes which love a dry garden bed. Another positive about a yucca garden is that it will be full of surprises. It's a specialist subject that is, actually, fascinating. But, crucially, no one wants to reach out and stroke a yucca. They have total respect in that way.

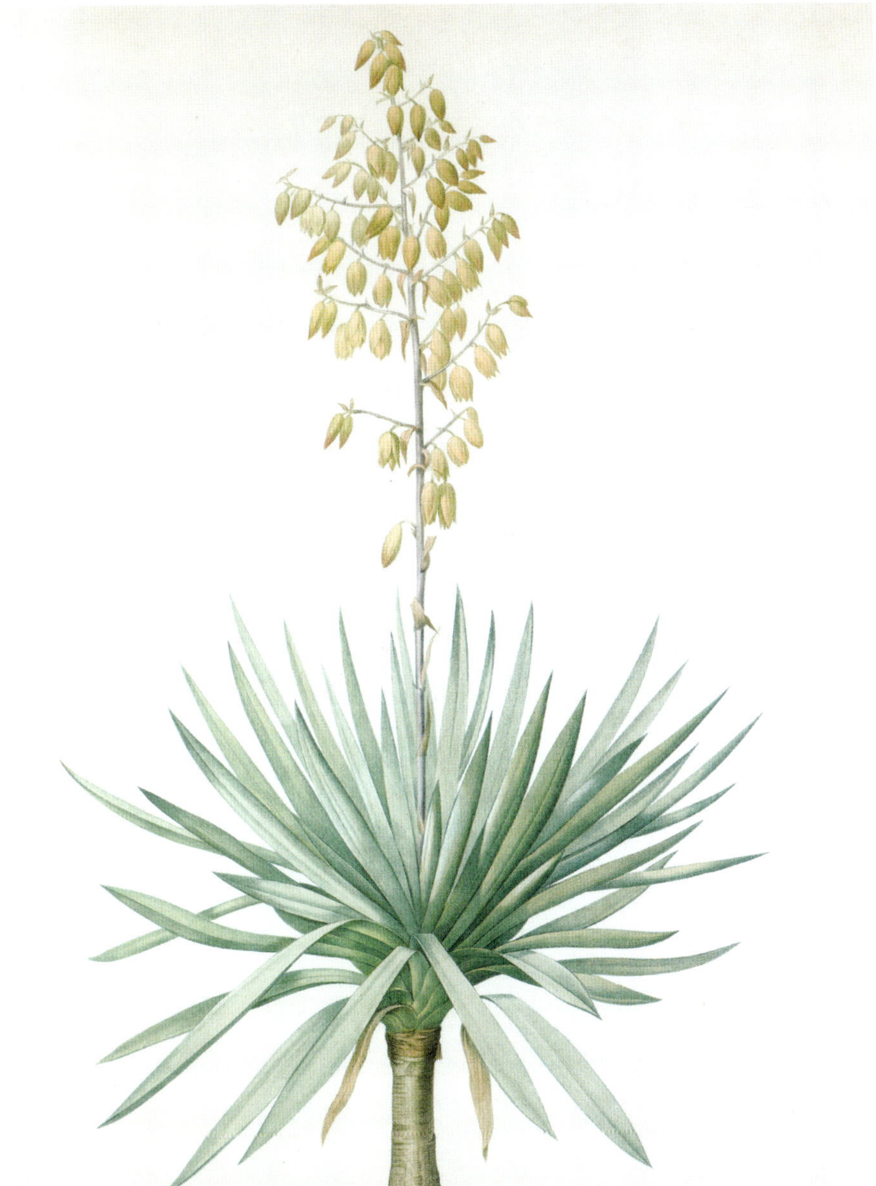

Yucca gloriosa by Pierre Joseph Redouté, from *Les Liliacées*, Vol. 6, 1807–16.

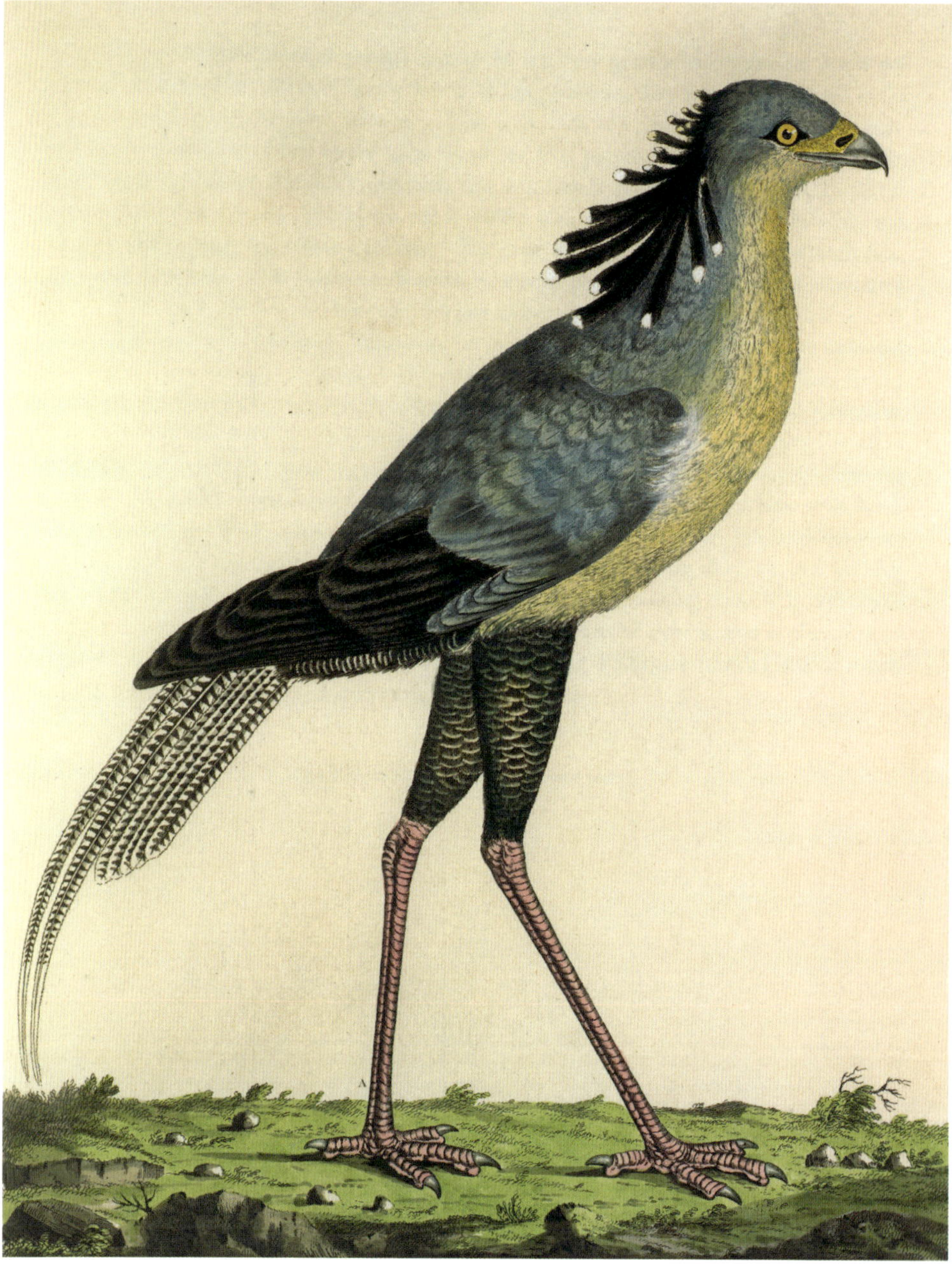

Secretary vulture, as drawn by George Shaw, from *Cimelia Physica: Figures of Rare and Curious Quadrupeds, Birds, etc, Together with Several of the Most Elegant Plants*, 1796.

You'd do worse than become a vulture for horticulture

Making money, obsessed with

There's a very succinct way to get over an obsession with money and no one put it better than an old-time American vaudeville comedian and singer named Jimmy Durante. His nickname was The Great Schnozzola, a reference to his nose, a subject that he rarely tired of. He was at the height of his popularity in the 1950s when he recorded the album *In Person*. There, amid such songs as 'It's My Nose's Birthday' and 'I'll Do the Strut-Away in My Cutaway', is a strangely wise song called 'I'm A Vulture for Horticulture'.

It's almost spooky how this song, written by Sid Kuller and Lee Wainer, and released in 1950, summed up what we now know are the phenomenal health and well-being benefits of getting out into the garden. One day you're obsessed with money and the next you are inspired to create your own Garden of Eden where every bud is your buddy. It's hard not to be persuaded or indeed influenced, and so here's a Durante-inspired fairytale of money and dirt which is not, of course, the same thing as dirty money.

Our man (though it could just as easily be a woman) is called Matt (short for materialistic) and money is everything to him. One day, as he sits idly looking out of a window, musing on a ludicrously high profit figure he is chasing, he sees a honey bee buzzing around a window box, in pursuit of some nectar. Something in his mind just switches on in that moment. That bee looked happy – and busy.

It helps to be a little bit rich, of course, and so Matt buys a little plot of land and soon he can be found tiptoeing through his very own tulips. He grows roses and lilies, daisies and dahlias. He plants apple and pear trees. He is a vulture for horticulture, but he doesn't stop there. He gets his own beehive. He still makes money but now he (and his bees) also make honey and what he likes to think about is his flower patch. His life is rich but not in the same way.

To fight the desire, consider the case of Miss Ellen Willmott

Shoplift, desire to

There's theft and then there's ruin, and the story of brilliant horticulturist Miss Ellen Willmott serves as a lesson to anyone who is tempted. She was born in 1858 with not so much a silver spoon in her mouth as a silver trowel in her hand. Her home at Warley Place in Essex became, under her command, the must-see garden that attracted the great, the good and the seriously serious horticulturist. She was a genius when it came to plants but life was another story. She was known to pack a pistol and booby-trapped her bulb fields to deter thieves.

But it's not bulbs that Ellen Willmott was after when she visited the 'Veiling and Scarf' department at the Galeries Lafayette department store on London's Regent Street in February 1927. When she left the store, she was arrested for shoplifting a black and red scarf (value 13s 6d). As her biographer Sandra Lawrence tells the story, Willmott insisted it was a mistake, but her protests went unheeded, possibly because at the time the store had been hit by a spate of shoplifting by a gang called the Forty Elephants (related to the infamous Elephant & Castle mob and led by Diamond Annie). Willmott immediately demanded a phone call and, when the store realized she was ringing Queen Mary (as you do), they offered to drop the matter.

Willmott, notoriously prickly and furious by now, insisted on going to jail for a night and then on to trial. She revelled in her acquittal, so much so that she subsequently decided to sue the store itself. This provided another orgy of gory details of her eccentric existence (Miss Haversham comes to mind) to be chewed over by the press and public. Willmott may have won (though we'll never really know if that unpaid-for scarf was just a mistake), but her reputation was lost. She became renowned as a grade-A grump who secretly seed-bombed other gardeners with the extremely prickly *Eryngium giganteum,* which is now known as 'Miss Willmott's Ghost'. She died, almost broke, in 1934.

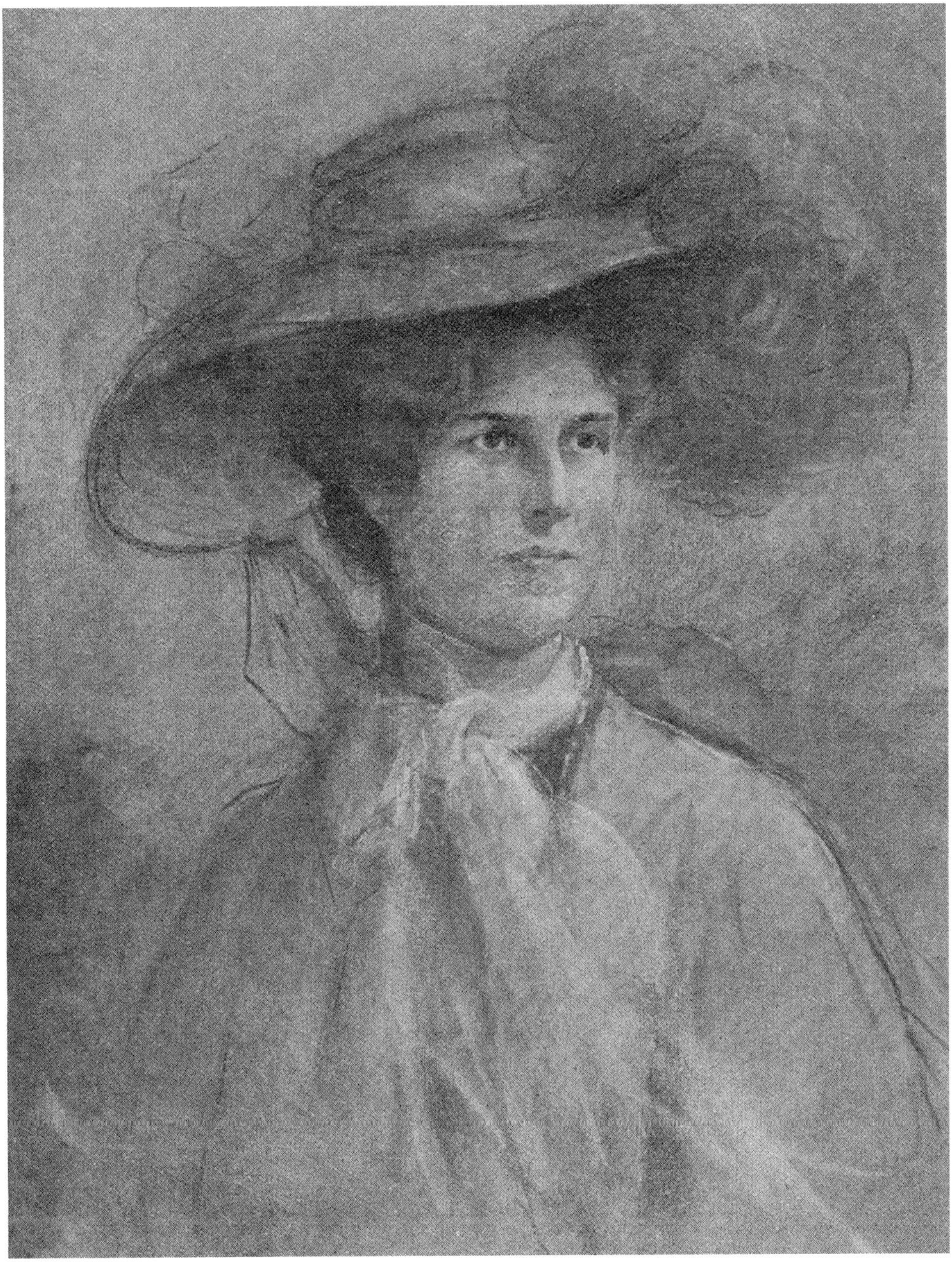

English horticulturist Miss Ellen Willmott, pastel portrait by Rosina Mantovani Gutti, as featured in *The Garden*, December 1907.

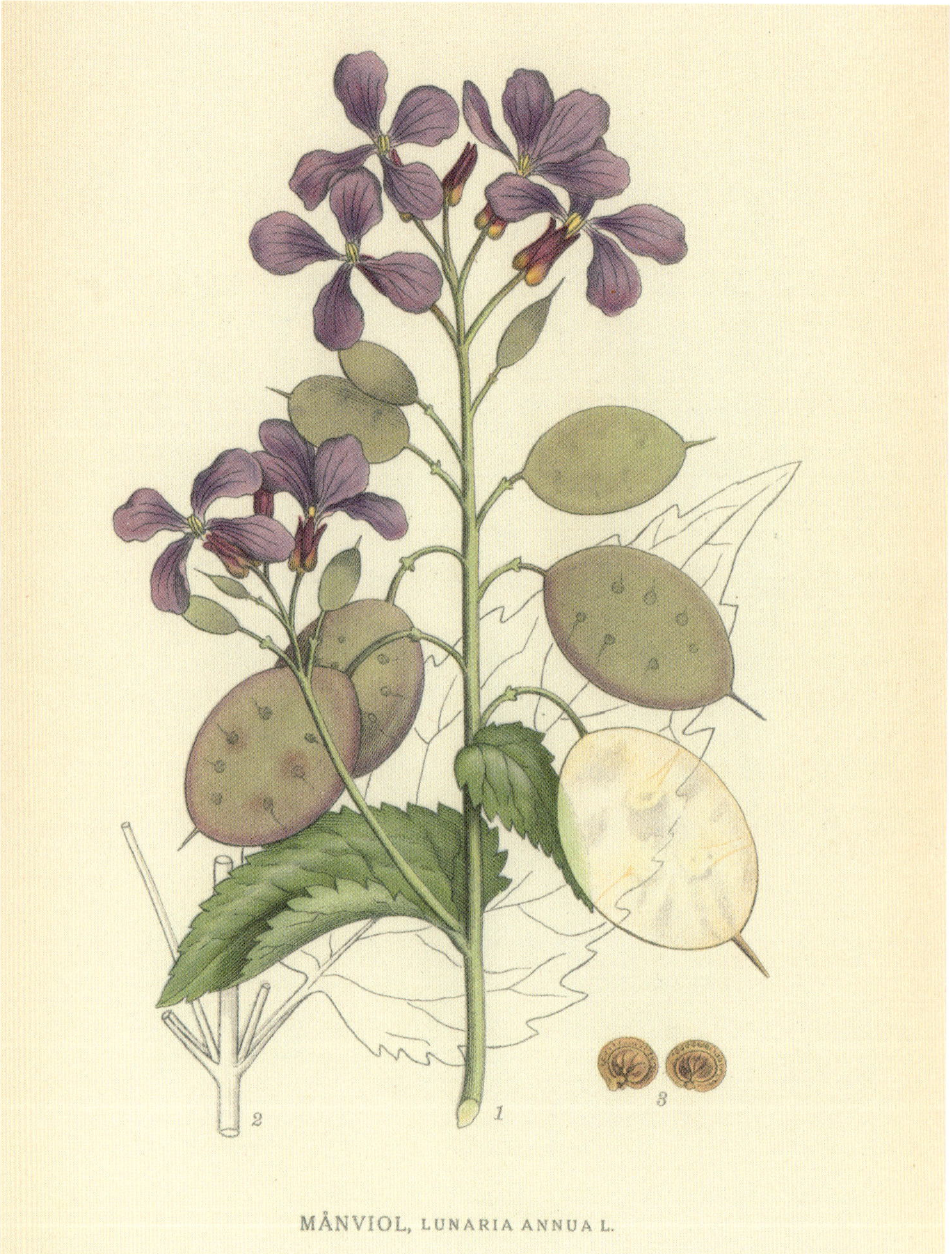

Honesty (*Lunaria annua*) by Carl Axel Lindman, from *Bilder ur Nordens Flora*, 1922.

It's all about making your money grow

Taxes, fear of

The fear of taxes is real and possibly more prevalent than a fear of death (see *Death, Fear of*, page 66). In the US, nearly one in three people say that even the thought of filing taxes makes them want to cry. People in the UK probably cry less than Americans anyway, but at least half of Britons dread the very thought of filing taxes. So, yes, taxes are taxing and the fear of them going up is even more widespread than the fear of filing them.

The garden cure is obvious. We all need to grow some money. It's often said that money doesn't grow on trees, though whoever said that wasn't entirely accurate. Some of the earliest banknotes in the world began life as plants: for instance, banknotes from China during the reign of Hongwu in 1368–98 were printed on paper made from the bark of the mulberry tree. Plus, plenty of trees produce valuable commodities (cocoa, coffee, rubber, palm oil, nuts and, last but never least, avocados) that bring in shedloads. Don't forget those plants/trees, such as *Crassula ovata* (aka the jade plant), which bring good luck. The Chinese practice of feng shui advises that every home or office should have one in its far left corner ('the wealth corner') to bring good fortune.

Trees, however, are large and may not fit into every garden (or indeed wealth corner). In this case, the easiest way to grow money is by sowing the seeds of *Lunaria annua*. This is commonly called honesty (also helpful when it comes to taxes) because its spring flowers, which can be white, pink or lavender, then fade into translucent discs called 'siliques'. These resemble coins and that is why *Lunaria* is also called 'moneywort' or the 'money plant'. It's a very generous plant, needing no encouragement to self-seed. This is welcome because taxes are fraught enough without worrying about how to grow money.

There's a perfectly dirty way to divert yourself from that phone

Doomscrolling, addiction to

It's a familiar scenario. You are supposed to be doing something else entirely – getting ready for work, going to sleep, cooking, cleaning, reading a book, combatting climate change, solving global problems. Instead you are sitting (or possibly lying, there is no prescribed position) and looking at your mobile phone, scrolling through headlines, apps, news feeds, notifications and just general stuff. 'Oh, just one more,' you say, looking at the clock which, irritatingly, is insisting on ticking away. But it's never just one more, is it? That's the problem with doomscrolling. It's a compulsion to read the next headline, then the next and the next. It makes you feel bad but you still keep scrolling.

There is no shortage of advice on how to tackle this unhealthy addiction. Top tips include setting boundaries, creating 'screen-free zones' and invoking the five-second rule which is, when you have a desire to scroll, to count to five first. Not sure that last one works at all, actually, but then, given the pervasive nature of doomscrolling, we aren't sure if any of the ideas work. Here's one that should. Let's try something far more fun that was put beautifully by Joni Mitchell in her 1970 song 'Woodstock' when she told us we were stardust and that we had to get ourselves back to the garden.

Yes, we do need to do exactly that. The garden should be a screen-free zone for many reasons. It's often hard to see the screen in the sunlight/rain/wind. You are probably without your glasses (or are wearing them on your head). It's dangerous to have your phone in your back pocket as it could fall out and be 'planted'. This is why it's so easy to lose your phone in the garden and so much better to leave it inside the house. Plus, in the garden, you are busy doing other things.

The garden cure for doomscrolling is weeding. This could include weeding of all kinds, but one treatment, in particular, has been found to be effective and that is weeding couch grass (*Elymus repens*) in a large perennial flower bed. If you are lucky enough to live in a part of the world without couch (pronounced 'cooch') grass, then rejoice and replace it with any weed that is pervasive and spreads through its roots/rhizomes.

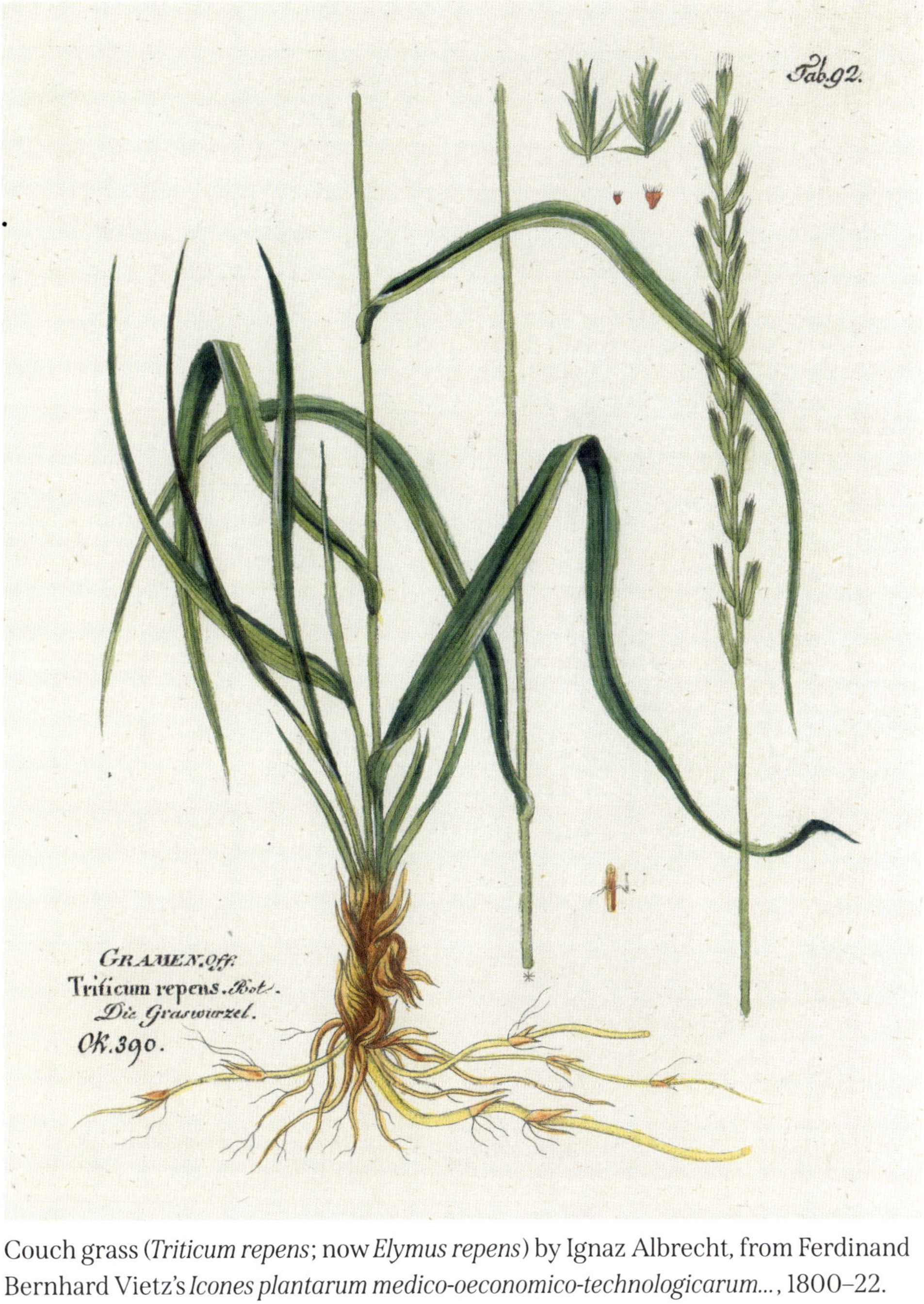

Couch grass (*Triticum repens*; now *Elymus repens*) by Ignaz Albrecht, from Ferdinand Bernhard Vietz's *Icones plantarum medico-oeconomico-technologicarum...*, 1800–22.

It's a war and you must be prepared. You will need gloves, a trowel, a large spade, a largish garden waste container (a trug is far too small). Ideally, you will be wearing 'gardening clothes' – in other words, clothes that are already dirty. You may want one of those colourful kneelers, though this is not really a kneeling job as it goes on for too long. Most of us, when we are weeding and not doomscrolling, end up sitting in the dirt.

Couch grass looks likc any innocent grass on the surface. All its nefarious activities take place underground. It has thin little white feeding roots. They are not a major issue. Your true enemy is the network of yellowish/brownish/whitish rhizomes that it uses to spread. You must remove every trace of these rhizomes. Even one tiny piece will, in time, infest the entire bed again.

Weeding couch grass can be as long as a piece of string or, in this case, rhizome. You see a blade of grass, dig down, follow the yellowish rhizome, then use the trowel, creating a trough as you follow it, sometimes for some way, to another tiny bit of green grass. Then you repeat. And repeat. You will encounter other weeds along the way, which may need removal, but don't allow yourself to forget the true enemy. It has been known for those involved in a war against this weed to spend hours on the battleground, but you are allowed breaks, to stop and just sit, appreciating the flowers, plants, sky, air. Avoid the house (and the phone) on your break as your shoes/trousers/etc. are all quite dirty. Besides, you don't want any distractions. Time no longer seems to matter as you follow yet another tough yellowish root/rhizome.

It's not just one battle but a series of battles over a long period of time. Weeds are amazingly prolific and resilient. You need to be exactly that too. You must stay alert. You can't do that if you're doomscrolling. Soon, you will find that the desire to doomscroll has been replaced by the desire to weed. You will feel better being outside in the fresh air, seeing the garden from the ground up, watching the bees and butterflies, as you continue to wage the battle. Will you win? That's the question that keeps you down and dirty, weeding away.

The three sisters are both a planting plan and a life lesson

Cooperation, longing for

There are many Native American legends about the three sisters, and this version is from the Iroquois (or Haudenosaunee as they are sometimes called) in upstate New York. Sky Woman is the mother of all humanity and she had a daughter who died in childbirth. From her grave, three plant sisters grew. One was tall with long, yellow hair and wore pale green. The next sister, who loved to hug and cling to her bigger sister, had a yellowish-green dress dotted with flowers. The third sister was so young that she could only crawl on the ground and circle the others' ankles. They were devoted to each other and, together, they fed the sons of Sky Woman's daughter and then, all of the world. They depended on each other absolutely and never wanted to be separated.

This may indeed be a story about corn (tall and willowy), beans (clingy and flowerful) and squash (low growing with large leaves) and how they served one another. Corn provided the structure that the beans depended on and the squash leaves shaded the ground, allowing the soil to remain moist. We now also know that the beans captured nitrogen from the air, releasing some into the soil, which would have fed the nitrogen-hungry corn.

It's a story about unity and love and how, if you find the right partners in an endeavour or, indeed, life, everyone can win. As a legend, it's life-affirming. As a planting plan, it's genius. As a metaphor, it's inspirational. It's handy to think about if you are stuck with a problem, and looking for a solution, to ask yourself: how would the three sisters work this out?

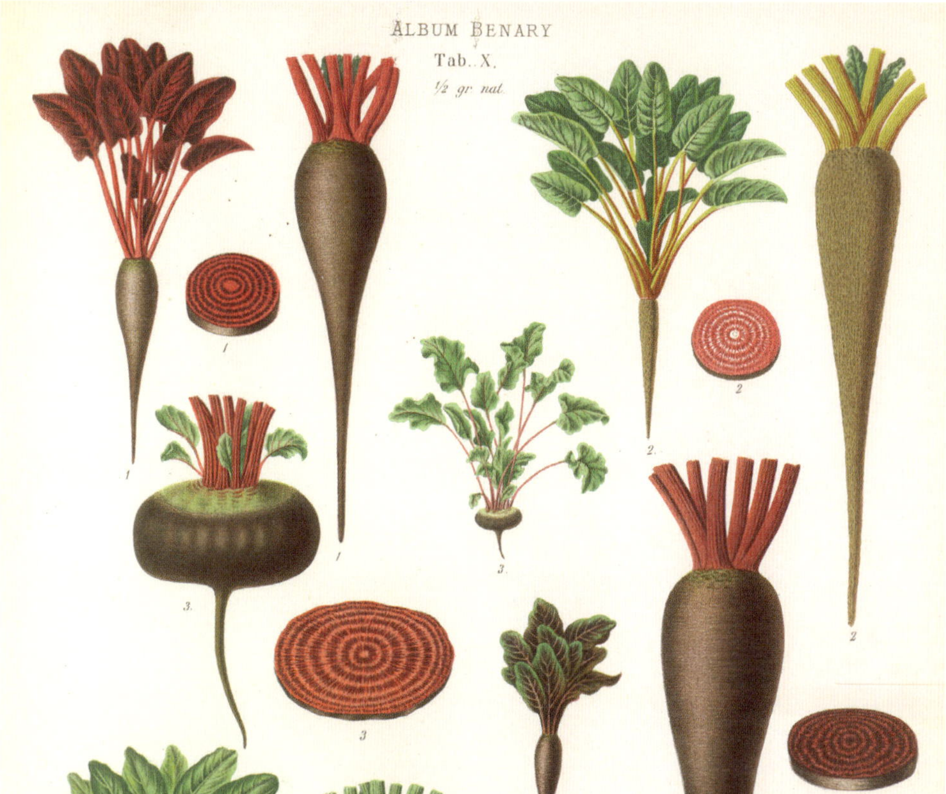

Beets by Ernst Benary, from *Album Benary*, 1876.

Sick of having to drive to the supermarket for fresh veg

Fresh vegetables, need for

Ron Finley lives in ultra-urban South Central Los Angeles and one day in 2010 he just decided he had had enough. 'I got tired of driving 45 minutes round trip to get an apple that wasn't impregnated with pesticides,' he says. Finley walked outside his home and surveyed the scene. He swept away the litter on the 'parkway', a strip of city land between kerb and sidewalk, in front of his house. He got some compost and began to plant a vegetable garden. It wasn't just any old veg. In addition to the usual crops, there was kale, pumpkin, sunflowers and a banana tree. But, because there is always at least one naysayer in every city block, one of his neighbours complained and the city promptly issued him with a citation and then a warrant for his arrest for obstructing sidewalks and kerbs. Finley credits that neighbour with what happened next. 'Embrace your haters because they make you famous,' he says.

Finley fought the citation and, boosted by a petition and an article in the *Los Angeles Times*, got the law changed. Now those litter-strewn 'parkway' plots, 45m (150ft) by 3m (10ft), could become gardens. And they did. That is how Finley, the self-styled 'Gangsta Gardener', became the father of an urban food forest revolution, with a global following and a Ted talk to boot. As part of the Ron Finley Project, based in South Central, he has led countless workshops with one message: food is the problem and food the solution.

'It all starts with one seed,' he says. 'Trust the powers and the magic and the alchemy that we have in connection to the planet.' He is a man who talks in inspirational sentences that often feel like slogans, such as 'If you want to get grounded, you touch the ground.' How do you go from a man who just wanted a nice apple to global gangsta gardener? 'When that opportunity comes, you take it. You go over the wall, through the wall, around the wall... You seize the day, or the day crushes you.' The message: plant a seed and anything can happen.

Get yourself to the garden and grow

Prison, finding yourself inside

Rikers Island is one of the most notorious prisons in the world, its dystopian landscape featuring a collection of low jail blocks and high razor wire. It is the largest prison in New York, housing its most violent criminals, but here – on this island in the East River between the Bronx and Queens – there is also something lush and green and beautiful. The Horticultural Society of New York (or The Hort, as it is called), in partnership with the city, has created seven gardens. The programme, called 'The GreenHouse', began in the late 1980s, started by a single volunteer. Its success, amid a culture of brutality and rampant violence, is both startling and inspiring. A 2008 study showed that inmates who garden have a 40 per cent less chance of reconviction and these results are similar in other studies.

The Hort is a force for good in general and their prison programme 'Therapeutic Horticulture' provides both training and, crucially, intern opportunities upon release. Prisoners work in the gardens four days a week, both learning about plants and landscaping basics, as well as growing edibles from seed and maintaining 98 raised beds and gardens that include cut flower beds, woodland, herbs and rose beds. The motivation behind the programme is nothing less than to help people, many with mental health issues and addictions, to change their lives for the better.

The overall thrust has been widely adopted with numerous programmes in multiple countries that train prisoners, and guards, in the basics of horticulture, as well as work with them to create gardens (including a garden at the RHS Chelsea Flower Show). The idea, tried and true, is that the prisoners are not only growing plants but also a new belief in themselves. As one prisoner told The Hort: 'When I lay in bed at night, I'm thinking of the garden – where should I plant this red hibiscus? Should I have put the grass somewhere else? Why on earth am I thinking of the garden at night? It just means so much to me!'

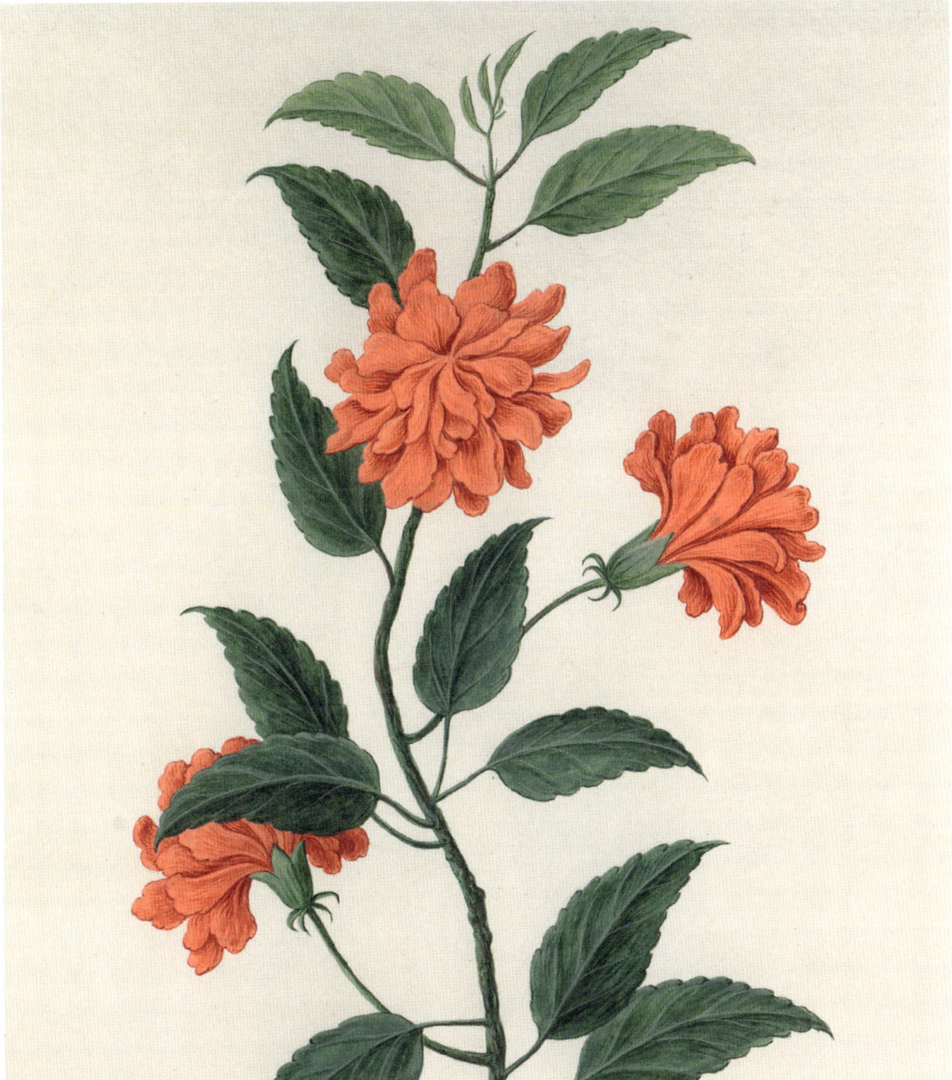

Chinese hibiscus (*Hibiscus × rosa-sinensis*), watercolour on paper (artist unknown) from *Règne Végétal*, Vol. 2, 1796.

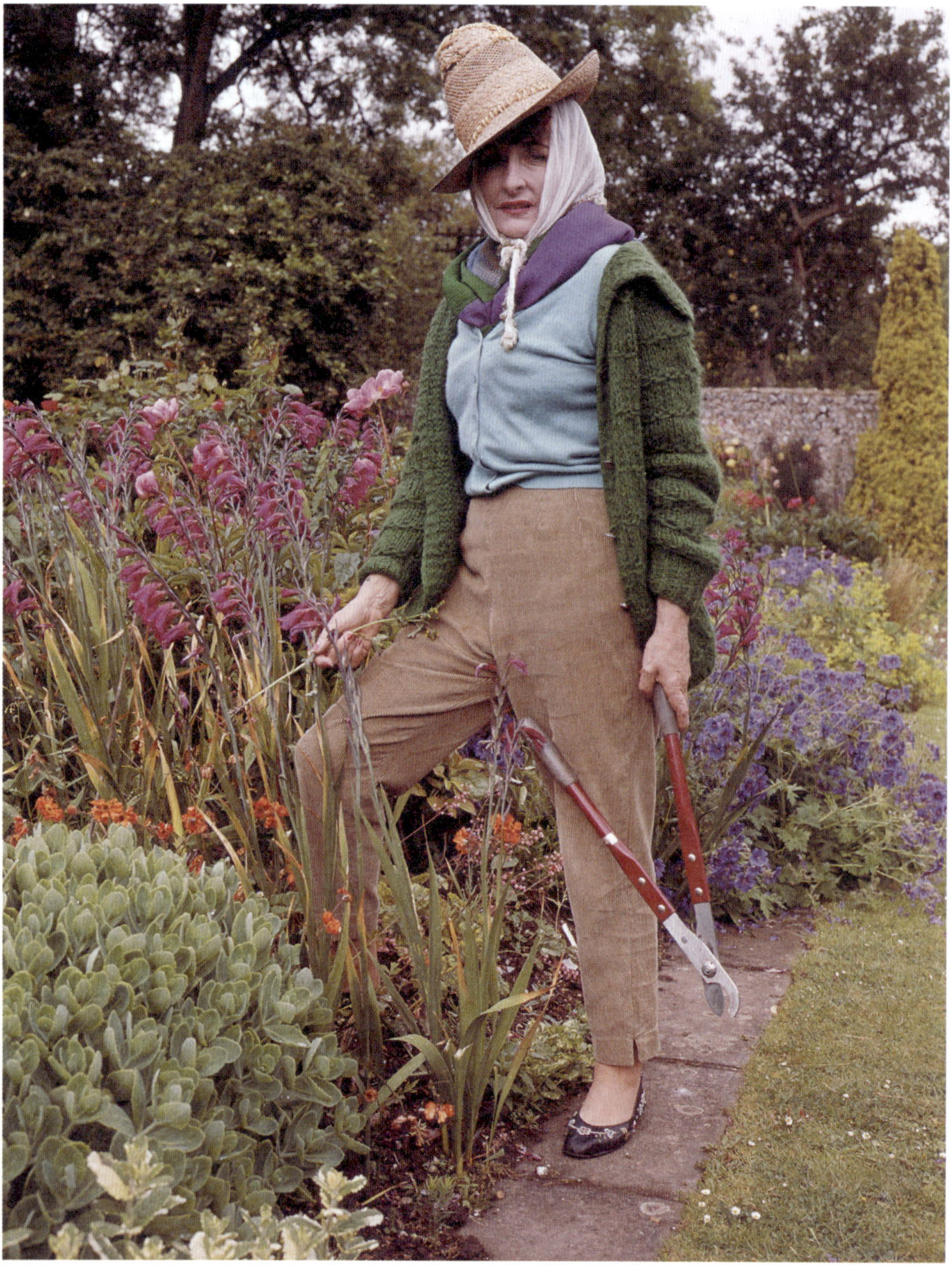

Lady Rhoda Birley tidying the garden at Charleston Manor, East Sussex, photographed by Valerie Finnis in the 1970s.

'The Three Ds' provide a strategy for seeing what to keep

Declutter, need to

We live in a world where the minimalist is a rare species. Most of us have too much stuff and a small industry of books/videos/media aimed at helping us to declutter has sprung up. The goal is to decide what to keep, give away or bin. Strategies include those with a geographical bent, called the ski slope, where you slalom this way and that, across a room, decluttering as you go. Then there's the number strategy (3, 5, 10 items per day, every day, and so on). There are also gurus such as Marie Kondo, who is all about having us hold up objects and decide whether they 'spark joy' in our innermost being.

The garden cure, which may indeed spark joy, especially when you are finished, is to take a lesson from the pruning guidebook. Pruning strategy is summed up neatly by the phrase: 'The Three Ds'. These are, in order, dead, diseased and damaged. First, you remove all dead areas from the shrub, pruning shoots down to the base or trunk. You then look for any sign of disease and remove those. Damaged includes any stems hurt by frost or drought, wind or, perhaps, foraging animals. You will also need to remove stems that cross each other. Your goal, in most cases, is to achieve an airy, well-spaced network of branches, with no crossing stems.

How does this relate to the fourth D (as in declutter)? For dead, read things that are no longer of any interest to you. The ski poles that you haven't used for 25 years, the cookbook that has never been opened, the dress that is two sizes too small. Get your virtual secateurs out and prune, prune, prune. Diseased includes any items that look tatty, broken, moth-eaten. The definition of 'damaged' is wider and includes evaluating anything 'crossing each other' or at odds in any way, as in too many pairs of trousers, wine glasses, coats, and such like. It really does help to think that you are pruning, not decluttering. Finally, step back from your work and decide what else needs to go for the shrub/home/wardrobe to be at its best. Then just do it.

You don't need to strew (but you can) to love sweet woodruff

Strew herbs, desire to

Do you ever have the desire to live in ages past? To retire from modern life and go 'off grid' and live life as it was in the 17th century? If so, you'll be very busy in the garden for those were the days when the garden provided food and drink, soap and medicine, flowers and fragrance. It is this last one that appeals here. The practice of strewing the floor with rushes and plants was a key part of home-coming preparations in the 17th century.

'Is supper ready? The house trimm'd, rushes strew'd, cobwebs swept...' asks the servant Grumio as his master Petruchio is on his way home in *The Taming of The Shrew* (Act IV, Scene I) by William Shakespeare. This was an era when rushes and sedges, combined with sweet-smelling herbs, were strewn on the floor, to protect clothes and to sweeten the air. Indeed, many plants with 'sweet' in their names – such as sweet flag (*Acorus calamus*) or sweet woodruff (*Galium odoratum*) – were all about making things smell nice during a time when things often didn't.

The tiny, delicate, white flowers of sweet woodruff that decorate the forest floor could be braided into garlands as well as added to the floor mix. It was also used as stuffing for beds. When dried, it smells of vanilla and newly mown hay, which is surely more delicious than any modern air freshener could ever be. Can't you just almost smell it now? How sweet it is.

'Strewing the floor with rushes and plants was a key part of home-coming preparations.'

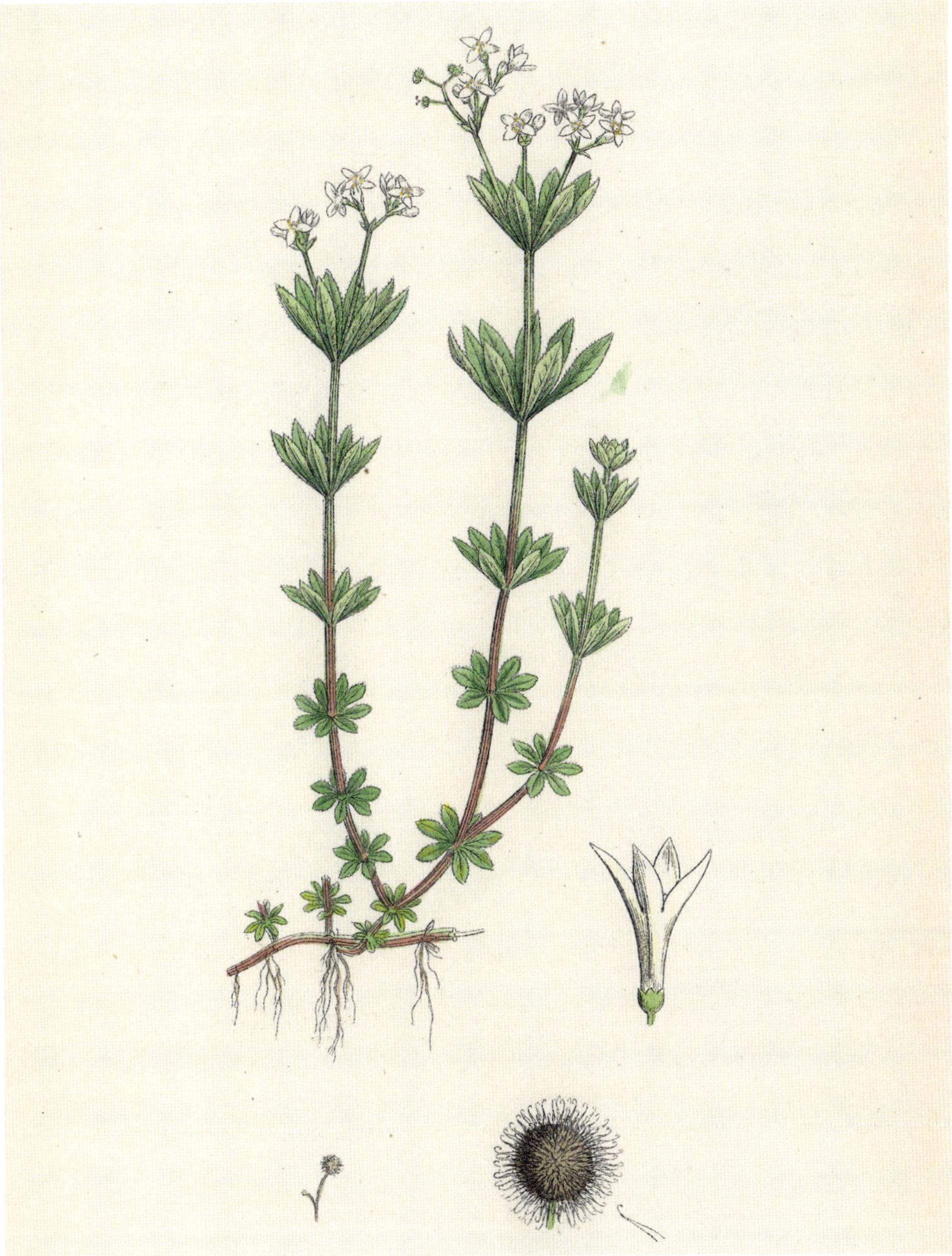

Sweet woodruff (*Galium odoratum*), from James Sowerby's *English Botany, or Coloured Figures of British Plants*, Vol. 4, 1863–1886.

An easy way to find a friend who demands nothing from you

Low-maintenance friends, seeking

Friends are, of course, wonderful to have, but you may feel that you already have enough. Some friends (the best ones) are no work at all, requiring little or nothing except what you want to give whenever you feel you have the time and/or inclination. Others can be high maintenance, requiring phone calls, texts, photo exchanges, letters and, in general, constant communication. This can be too much, sparking a yearning for a friend who simply exists and is happy to do so. The garden has a perfect cure for this in the form of the garden gnome.

This may set off alarm bells, particularly if you think garden gnomes are tacky, plasticky and generally tasteless creatures. But the truth about gnomes is that they have a fine ancestral history and they can come in almost any form. The Romans weren't averse to a small statue or two in the garden, and gnomes had their first proper outing during the Renaissance when they were seen as small (under one foot tall), magical figures who preferred their own company to anyone human. They've evolved from there and the garden gnomes we are most familiar with are descended from those created in Germany in the 1800s, which were often very small (15cm/6in) and seen as 'little folk' who could help on the farm or mines.

The oldest known gnome (don't say that too fast) is named Lampy and is the only survivor of a batch of 21 brought to England from Germany by Sir Charles Isham in 1874. The gnomes were styled as various types of workers, including blacksmiths and miners (some of whom were on strike, complete with signs), and were placed in groups in the magnificent rockery, 7.3m (24ft) high, at Lamport Hall, his home in Northamptonshire. Sir Charles,

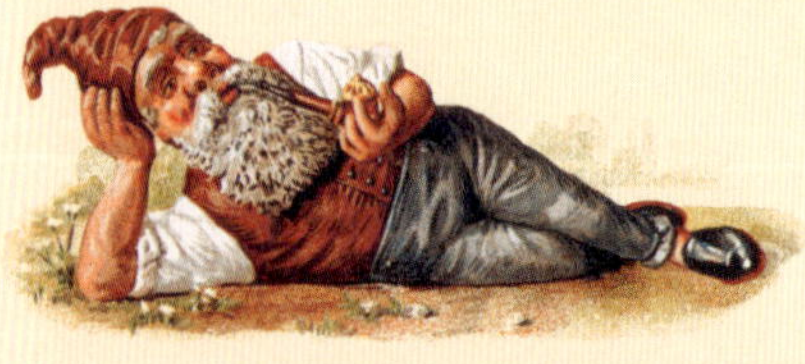

A selection of designs for garden gnomes from the German company Heissner, *c*.1910.

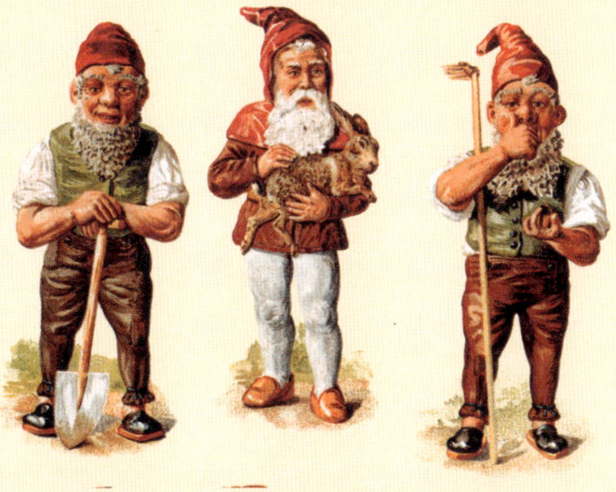

a spiritualist and rural improver, saw his diminutive gnomes (15cm/6in tall) as real. 'Had gnomes been imaginary creations,' he explained in 1884, 'they would not have been admitted into the Lamport Rockery. Although the nature of Gnomes is at present very obscure, it is, like all other occult phenomena, receiving attention throughout the world.'

The status of garden gnomes has waxed and waned over subsequent years, boosted in the 1930s by Snow White with her busy little miner friends named Doc, Grumpy, Happy, Bashful, Sleepy, Sneezy and Dopey. (They were called dwarfs but seen by most as gnomes.) There have also been travelling gnomes, perhaps the most famous of which is depicted in the film *Amelie* in which a stolen gnome travels around the world, being photographed in exotic locations. It's all a ruse to try and get Amelie's father to become less reclusive and to get out and travel the world.

If this all sounds rather high maintenance, you would be right. But the great thing about a garden gnome, or indeed multiple gnomes, is that they can simply just 'be'. They don't have to travel, work in mines or converse with Disney princess types. They can just stand, sit or lounge in your garden, ready to listen to you when and if you decide to speak to them. They are truly great friends: always there, never critical or demanding. There is, after all, no place like gnome.

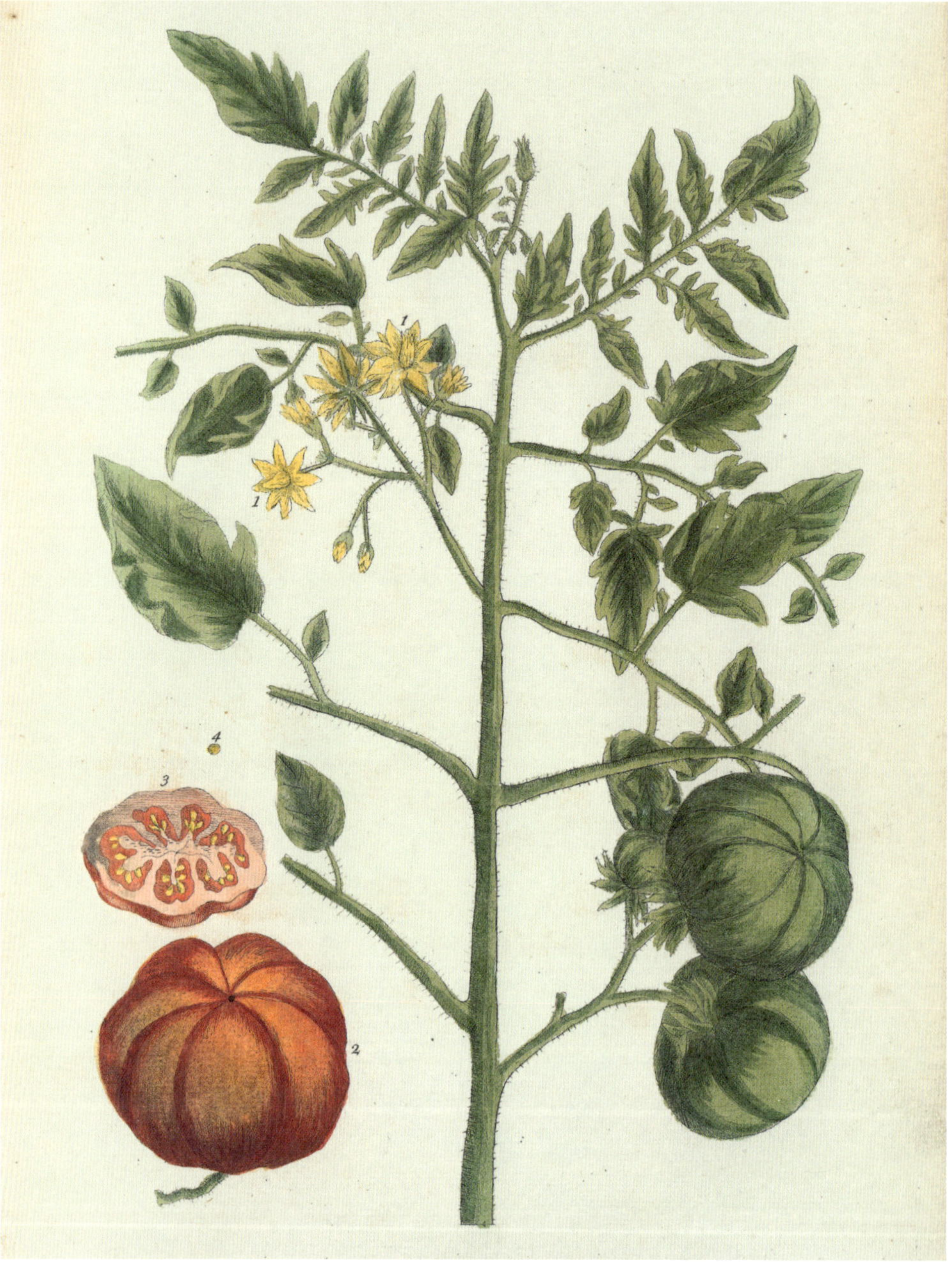

Tomato (*Solanum lycopersicum*), or love-apple, as described and drawn by Elizabeth Blackwell, from *A Curious Herbal*, Vol. 1, 1737.

All is not lost if you channel Elizabeth Blackwell

Married, to a scoundrel

If you suspect that you are married to a scoundrel, then take heart from the story of Elizabeth Blackwell, née Simpson, who was born in the City of London in 1699. You may already be wondering about this name as there is another EB who became the first female doctor. But our Elizabeth Blackwell lived more than a century earlier. She was not a doctor, of course, though her husband, Alexander, whom she married in 1733, seemed to think he was. On paper, Alexander was a bit of a catch. He came from a good Aberdeen family, his father was a senior figure in the Church of Scotland and principal of Marischal College. Alexander himself claimed to have graduated in medicine from Leiden.

Did Elizabeth wonder why someone who was a doctor, and one who claimed to have studied with the great Herman Boerhaave in Leiden, was now a proofreader for a printer in London? We don't know, but her husband managed to make things worse (a theme of his life) by pooh-poohing the requirement to do an apprenticeship before setting up as a printer himself. The print union wasn't impressed. The result was that two years after they were married, Alexander was sent as a bankrupt to debtor's prison.

Elizabeth, the daughter of a painter, had a lifelong love of drawing, but she must have had a seriously good business brain too because she came up with the idea of creating a 'herbal', to be used by apothecaries and doctors, drawing plants from real life. These included the newly exotic ones coming in from around the world, including coffee, nutmeg, cinnamon and the love-apple, now known (and still much loved) as the tomato. London's Chelsea Physic Garden as well as prominent doctors backed her (amazing in itself) and over the next two years she produced a total of 500 images for the herbal. She engraved them in copper herself and then personally hand-coloured them. She was a one-woman illustration factory, rushing back and forth to prison where Alexander provided the text.

It worked! She managed to pay off Alexander's debts and the book, with the somewhat longish title *A Curious Herbal containing five hundred cuts of the most useful plants, which are now used in the practice of physick, to which is added a short description of ye plants and their common uses in physick* was hailed as a success. Alexander emerged from prison in 1737 and Elizabeth probably sighed with relief. Their first son died shortly after birth and now there was a daughter. Perhaps she imagined a settled family life ahead.

Alexander had other ideas. He turned his talents to fertilizing methods and ended up moving to Sweden in 1742 (on his own) to try his luck there. Somehow he managed to find royal favour (including a salary and pension) with King Frederick I. Meanwhile Elizabeth, back in London, is said to have kept sending him money from the herbal.

But once a scoundrel, always a scoundrel. Amazingly, Alexander was appointed as personal physician to the King but, in 1747, was put on trial for treason, having become a player in political intrigue. He was beheaded, providing a final jovial moment when he put his head on the wrong side of the block, saying he had never been beheaded before. Elizabeth lived out the rest of her life in obscurity in London. Still, she is now very famous indeed, her work celebrated and adored. Just think: if her husband hadn't been a scoundrel, there would never have been a herbal or any fame or fortune.

'Once a scoundrel, always a scoundrel.'

It may make you feel better to know you aren't an aphid

Self-pity, wallowing in

It's easy to give in to self-pity in modern life. You know that feeling where, after a particularly cruel day, you see yourself as a victim of not only that day but of all days. To be clear, this is not a reference to a real trauma but refers to a series of events which, by themselves, are unimportant but, when taken together in the wrong frame of mind, could be seen as a plot against you. The garden is not against self-pity because it doesn't judge. If you are feeling very sorry for yourself, then your first move should be to get out to the garden.

While you are there, your eye may alight on a rose bush, and on the leaves you may see some green or black specks. These are aphids (there are many types and they belong to the family Aphididae) and, if it's a warm day, they'll be out and about more than usual. Frankly, though, who would be an aphid? Their life cycle has a Cinderella-like drudgery to it (without the slipper or the Prince Charming). In the spring, the overwintering eggs hatch into wingless female nymphs which are already pregnant. It's asexual reproduction (that is, cloning), and they give live birth to more wingless females (who are themselves already pregnant). It would be a horror film if anyone really cared about them as much as we do roses. One adult female aphid can give birth to up to 80 offspring, and a new aphid can become a mother in as few as seven days.

What a reproductive treadmill it is, and the point here is that there's no escape. Aphids can't take holidays or get divorced. They are trapped in an endless cycle of pregnancy and birth. Now that's pitiful and, though this is not a sure-fire cure, it may make you feel better to know that things would be definitely worse if you were an aphid.

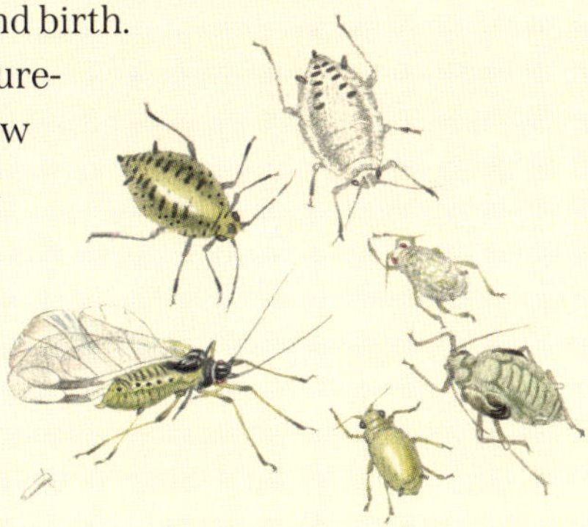

Aphids by George Bowdler Buckton, from *Monograph of the British Aphides*, 1879–81.

It's been the cure for everything from malaria to worms

Medicinal alcohol, popularity of

There is almost no alcoholic drink that has not, at some point, been considered medicinal. 'To your health!' people say, raising a glass of whisky or rum or, indeed, almost anything. This, even though alcohol is actually a poison that is classified, along with tobacco and asbestos, as a Group One Carcinogen by the World Health Organization. It's an unusual kind of 'medicine' that affects the brain's memory, balance and speech capacities but, hey, that may just be the drink talking. A drink or two can certainly mask whatever is troubling you, at least for a time, as it increases the 'happy hormone' dopamine in our brains until it all crashes into clumsiness, nausea and dehydration.

The history of alcohol is as old as plants. It's entirely possible that the grapes in the Garden of Eden (unspecified variety) may have naturally fermented, leading to all kinds of chaos. The garden, in the case of alcohol, is not so much the cure as the problem. Without plants, we'd all have a very tiny drinks cupboard. It all begins with photosynthesis in which sunlight and oxygen are used to create carbon dioxide and sugar. Add yeast to sugar and you get alcohol. Sugar cane makes rum, grapes become wine, potatoes produce vodka, and barley/wheat make whisky, gin, more vodka and beer. That's only the starter list. Here then are a few of the 'cures':

Absinthe: Lethally high alcohol content (up to 80% ABV). Made from wormwood (*Artemisia absinthium*), as well as green anise and sweet fennel. Invented by Dr Pierre Ordinaire during the French Revolution. It was called the 'green fairy' as too much led to hallucinations and madness, and was prescribed for the treatment of epilepsy, kidney stones, headaches and roundworms.

Gin and tonic: The first anti-malarial cure. The active ingredient here is quinine, from the bark of the cinchona tree (*Cinchona officinalis*), but it was so bitter that British soldiers in 18th-century India mixed it with sugar, gin (40–50% ABV) and lime to make it more palatable. The lime could be construed as a cure for scurvy. Tonic today doesn't contain enough quinine to cure anything.

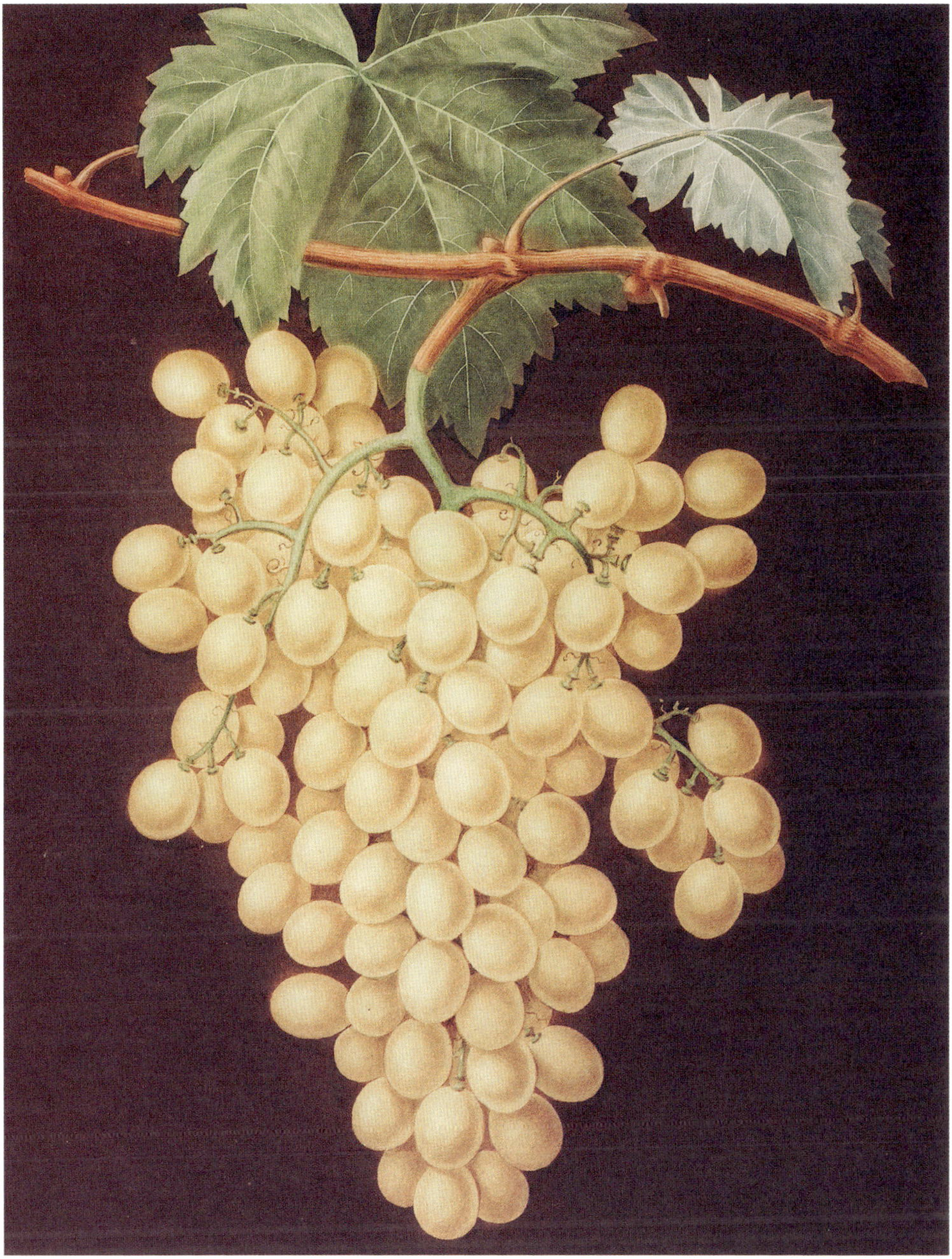

'Muscat of Alexandria' grapes by George Brookshaw, from *Pomona Britannica: or, a Collection of the Most Esteemed Fruits at Present Cultivated in this Country*, 1804–12.

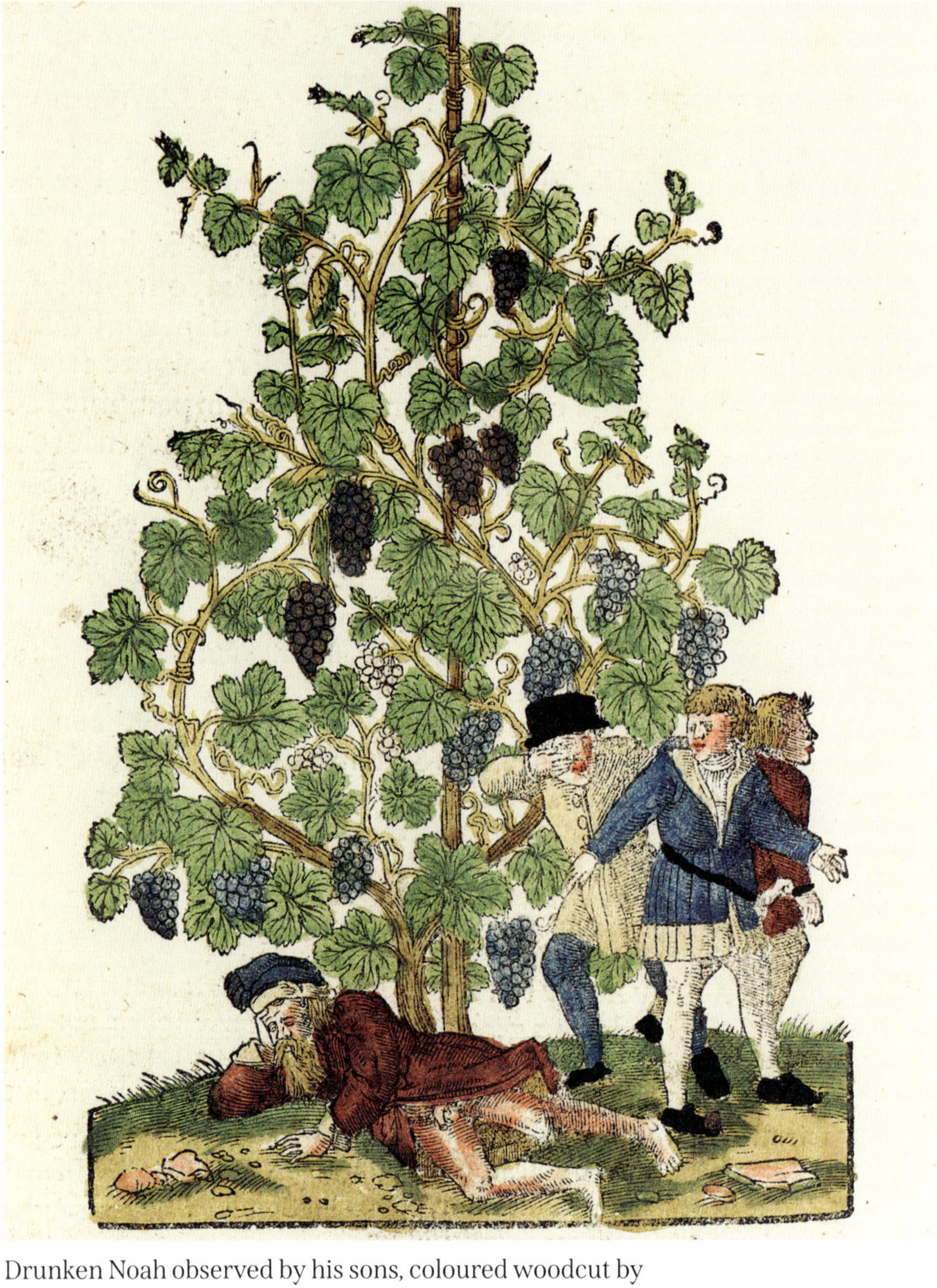

Drunken Noah observed by his sons, coloured woodcut by Hieronymus Bock, from *De stirpium Hieronymi Tragi*, 1552.

Aquavit: A Scandinavian spirit (about 40% ABV) from grain or potatoes, made since the 15th century. Herbs and botanicals include caraway seeds. Its name means 'water of life' and it was believed to ward off disease and old age. It was prescribed as a medicine against the Black Death. Legend reports that it can bring people back from the dead (unsourced).

Rum: Made from sugar cane (about 40% ABV) and viewed as a cure-all for many ailments, particularly by sailors from the 17th to 19th centuries. Used for scurvy, colds and sore throats ('hot toddy'), insomnia, insect bites/stings, and to clean wounds. It was also believed to ward off evil spirits.

Brandy: Made from fermented fruit, most often grapes, with a range of 30–60% ABV. It was prescribed for colds and flu, digestion, pain and heart issues. It was often seen as a resuscitation agent during the late 1800s and early 1900s. A paper by Henry Guly, partly funded by the Wellcome Foundation, on 'Medicinal Brandy' contains this pithy description of how brandy was referred to during the Heroic Age of Antarctic Exploration (1897–1922):

'For example [Edward] Wilson said of [Robert Falcon] Scott's first expedition: "No alcohol was taken on sledge journeys, except for a small can of brandy for emergencies"... Spirits other than brandy could be used: on the Belgian expedition, Amundsen 'gave Tollefsen a glass of cherry liqueur on the doctor's advice' for 'exhaustion, mixed with madness' but other spirits were thought less useful. Thus Bernacchi on the Southern Cross Expedition (1898–1900), in complaining that the expedition leader had consumed all the brandy, wrote in his diary: 'Unless the doctor has a bottle or so, we have not a drop of brandy at Cape Adair for medicinal purposes. On this occasion we were obliged to use whiskey. It is really scandalous.'

This last complaint illustrates perfectly one of the major problems with alcoholic 'medicinal' cures. They were prone to disappearing, almost by magic, leaving you with an empty cabinet.

What works if you've had too much medicinal alcohol?

A hangover, suffering from

There is no official cure for a hangover, but the garden has some ideas when it comes to this. After all, it is only right that the garden, having been responsible for the plants that produced the alcoholic drinks causing the hangover, can also produce some of the antidotes. It's going to be quite the concoction, if you put it all together. First, think coconut water. The fact it is water is a huge plus, as you will be dehydrated, but it's also full of electrolytes to recharge your body and can also help with headache and nausea. Tomato juice (no vodka) can also be an effective remedy. Of course, tomato juice also includes a lot of water and tomatoes contain beta-carotene, vitamins A and C, and the antioxidants lycopene and glutathione. In both these cases, you can pretreat the problem by drinking a glass before you go out.

By the way, this cure is not from the garden, but most of the world swears by a toastie and/or full English breakfast. Other (healthier) options are bananas (replenishing that potassium) and ginger (good for nausea). There's also milk thistle (*Silybum marianum*), a herbal remedy aimed at protecting the liver. Finally, and this will make for a very interesting breakfast addition, there is the humble artichoke (*Cynara cardunculus*), which is also a type of thistle, said to improve liver health and digestion. Cheers!

'There is no official cure for a hangover, but the garden has some ideas…'

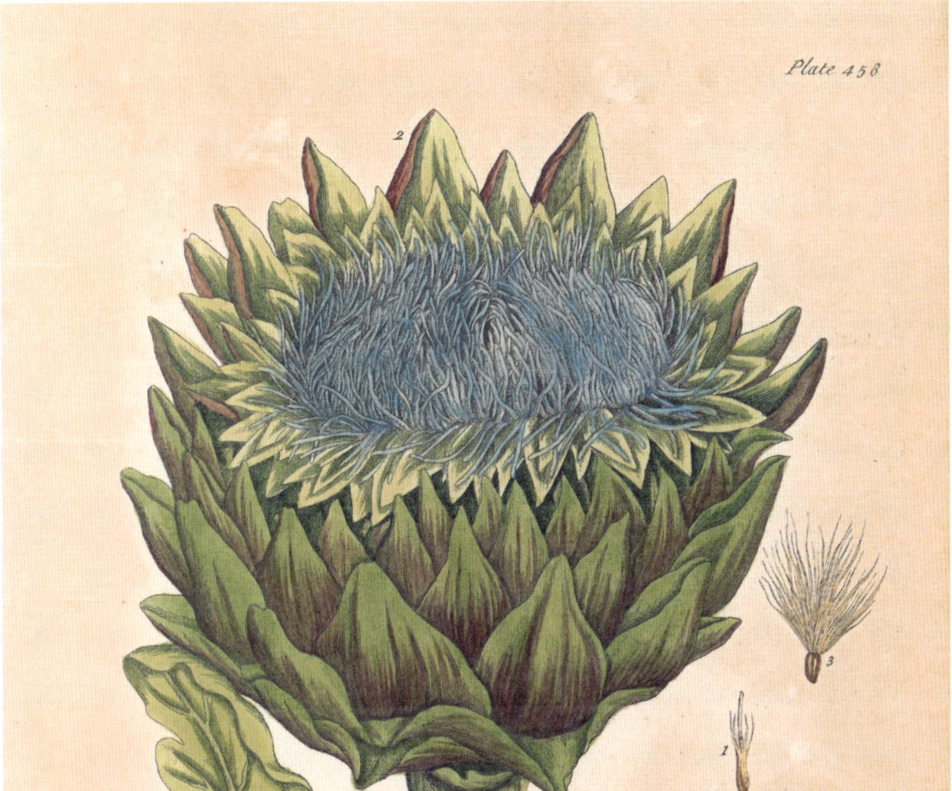

Artichoke (*Cynara cardunculus*) by Elizabeth Blackwell, from *A Curious Herbal*, Vol. 2, 1737–39.

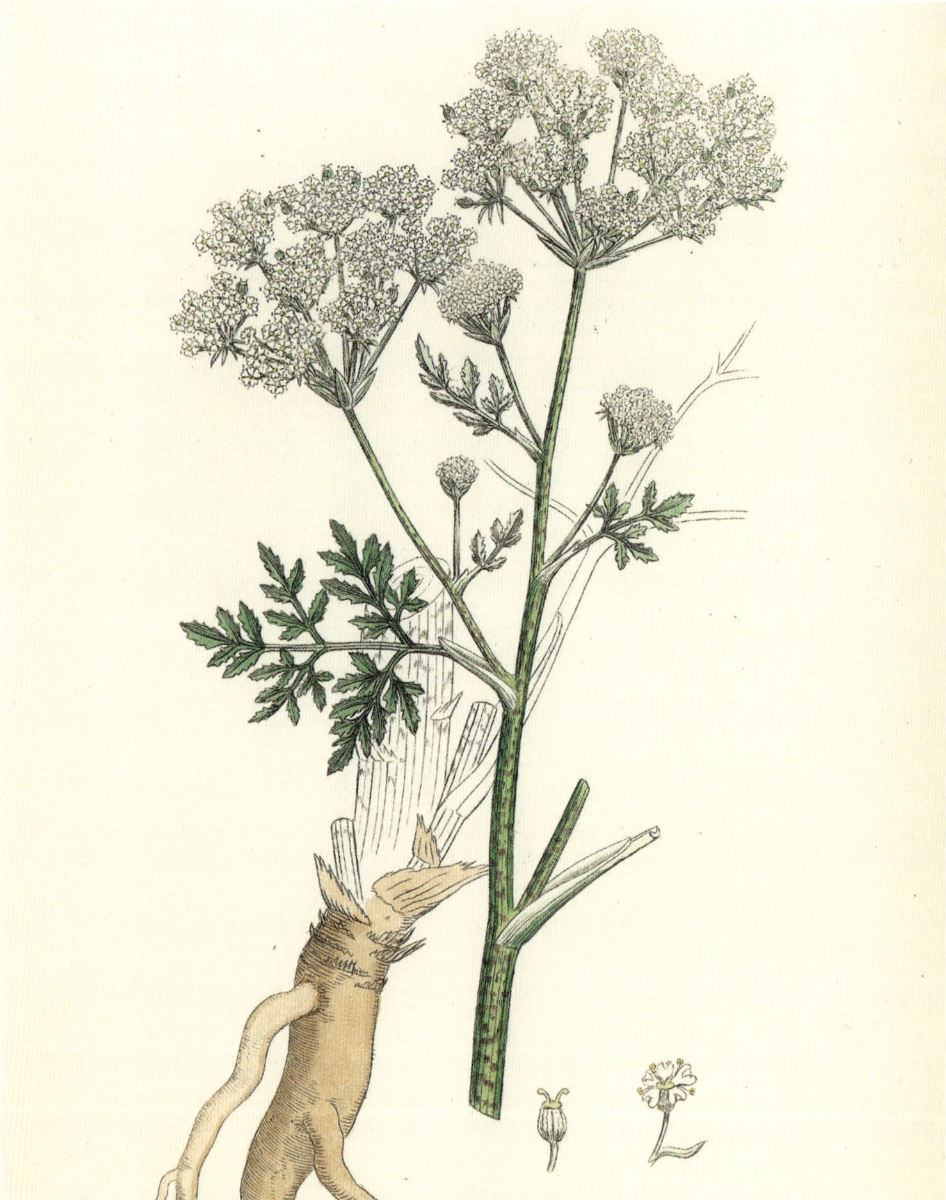

Hemlock (*Conium maculatum*) by James Sowerby, from James Edward Smith's *English Botany, or Coloured Figures of British Plants...*, Vol. 17, 1790–1814.

If you see murder in the garden, you know who to blame

Agatha Christie, too much

Do you sometimes wonder if you've read (or watched) too many Agatha Christie murder mysteries? Do you walk through a small English village and think, when you spy a rose-covered cottage, I wonder who's inside there, plotting to kill? You aren't alone. This is the legacy of the Queen of Crime. No one saw a garden quite the way Agatha Christie did. During the First World War, she had trained as an apothecary's assistant, and her Red Cross service card reveals that she did 3,400 hours in service. By the end of the war, she knew a great deal about poisons. 'Give me a decent bottle of poison,' she said, 'and I'll construct the perfect crime.' But she didn't really need a bottle at all. All Christie needed was a garden.

Her favourite murder weapon was poison and her favoured source of that were plants of one kind or another. *Digitalis*, or foxglove, was the killer in four cases. Aconite, from the roots of monk's hood (*Aconitum napellus*), aka wolf's bane, appears in two mysteries. Then there's hemlock (*Conium maculatum*), yew, deadly nightshade (*Atropa belladonna*) and yellow jasmine, now best known as jessamine (*Gelsemium sempervirens*). Another much used poison, strychnine, is found in the bark, seeds and roots of the strychnine tree, *Strychnos nux-vomica*. Then of course there's cyanide, which comes from the fruit stones of peaches, nectarines and other members of the *Prunus* genus.

It's not just murderous plants that are creepy. It's the other ones too, the sinister ones (Christie seemed to see plants almost as human.) In *Nemesis*, published when she was 81, she describes the grounds of a manor house in which a mound could be seen. Here a greenhouse had once stood but fell into disrepair, turning to rubble, with a certain plant all over it. 'A creeper well known when you want to hide or cover some rather ugly pieces of building in your garden. Polygonum it is called,' she writes. 'One of the quickest flowering shrubs which swallows and kills and dries up and gets rid of everything it grows over. It grows over everything. It is in a way a rather frightening plant. It has beautiful white flowers, it can look very lovely.' Chilling, yes? I think we know where the body was buried – under the *Polygonum* (or knotweed), of course.

Rustle up a botanical cocktail with someone else's name on it

James Bond, desire to be

Hello Mr Bond. This garden cure is for you. All Bond fans will know the name Vesper Lynd, the 'Bond girl' in Ian Fleming's 1953 classic *Casino Royale*. She's the one that Mr Bond first fell for. Her role may have been updated for the film in 2013 where she was a double agent (or was it triple?), but the crucial point is that Vesper was the one whom he fell for. Bond loved her enough to name 'his' cocktail after her. For him, that's a very deep commitment. Here's how he told the barman to make it in Chapter 7 of *Casino Royale*, which incidentally has the Bond-tastic title of 'Rouge et Noir':

3 parts gin (grain alcohol with essential juniper berries)
1 part vodka (Bond prefers vodka made from grain)
1 or ½ part Kina Lillet (wine-based aperitif flavoured with quinine from 'kina-kina' or chinchona tree bark). You can also use Lillet Blanc or Cocchi Americano.
Garnish is a large thin slice of lemon peel

You'll need the right glass, which we are told is a 'deep champagne goblet'. It must be ice-cold and shaken, not stirred (but you knew that). At the start of the book, this was Bond's special dry martini, but one without a name. It was while taking the beautiful, velvet-wearing Vesper Lynd (she was born on a 'stormy night', thus the Vesper, Latin for 'night') out to dinner in Chapter 7 that he decided. It was, he said, to be called 'The Vesper', adding: 'It sounds perfect and it's very appropriate to the violet hour when my cocktail will now be drunk all over the world.' He wasn't wrong.

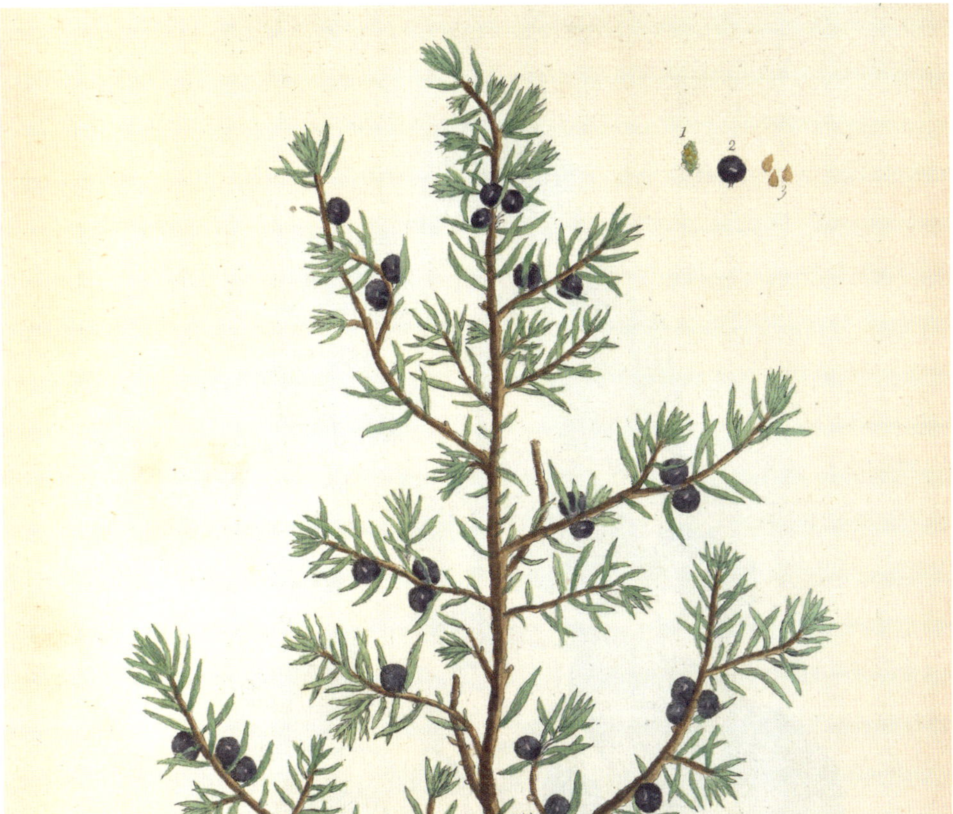

Juniper (*Juniperus communis*) by Elizabeth Blackwell, from *A Curious Herbal*, Vol. 1, 1737.

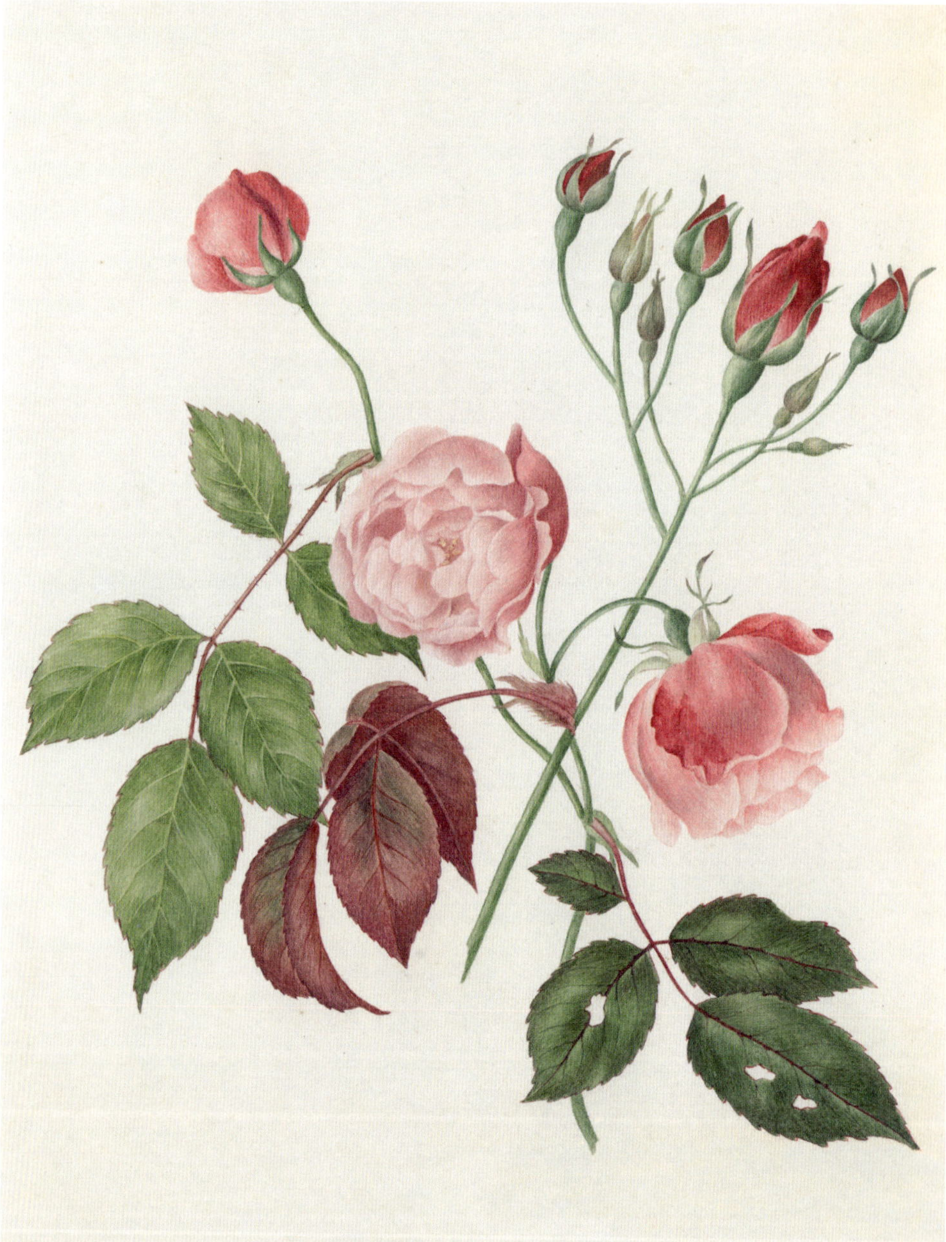

China Roses, watercolour on paper by Caroline Maria Applebee from Album 1, 1816.

Who needs a Porsche when you can find a growing obsession?

Mid-life crisis, looming

If you are of a certain age, which is most probably between 40 and 50, you may notice some changes taking place. You may suddenly dig out clothing from decades earlier, put it on and think: those thigh-high boots are still great! Or, perhaps, you have started thinking that leather is everyday wear. Other symptoms involve being attracted to a Porsche instead of your current Fiat Punto. Hair transplants might be a new interest. You may start to think that age is only a number and your destiny is to be forever 33. If so, get yourself out to the garden, pronto.

There are so very many projects in a garden that can easily take the place of a new Porsche. Is there anything more rewarding than succession plantings of wild tulips? Think of it, every corner of your patio could be bursting in various types and colours of tulips: there are 15 categories and, in all, more than 3,000 types. Pointy, ruffled, striped, bold, green, any other colour. You name it, there's a tulip out there somewhere that personifies it. Plus, you'll be saving money because *Tulpenwoede* or 'tulip madness', when people lost serious money over one bulb, occurred in the 1600s. In comparison, all things *Tulipa* are so much cheaper now.

If tulips do not appeal, then consider alpines or, gulp, carnivorous plants. Take up bonsai or orchids. Remember, it's never too late to develop a new obsession or, if you prefer the word, hobby. Take the story of Samuel Reynolds Hole, a vicar from Nottinghamshire who, in the late 1880s became Dean of Rochester in Kent. But the church was not enough for Hole who was, when he was in his forties, asked to judge a rose contest, though he knew not why (having no roses). He went, judged, fell in love with them and ordered a dozen immediately. He didn't stop there either: 'Year by year my enthusiasm increased... my roses multiplied from a dozen to a score, a score to a hundred, a hundred to a thousand, from one to five thousand trees.' All in all, so much nicer in every way than a Porsche.

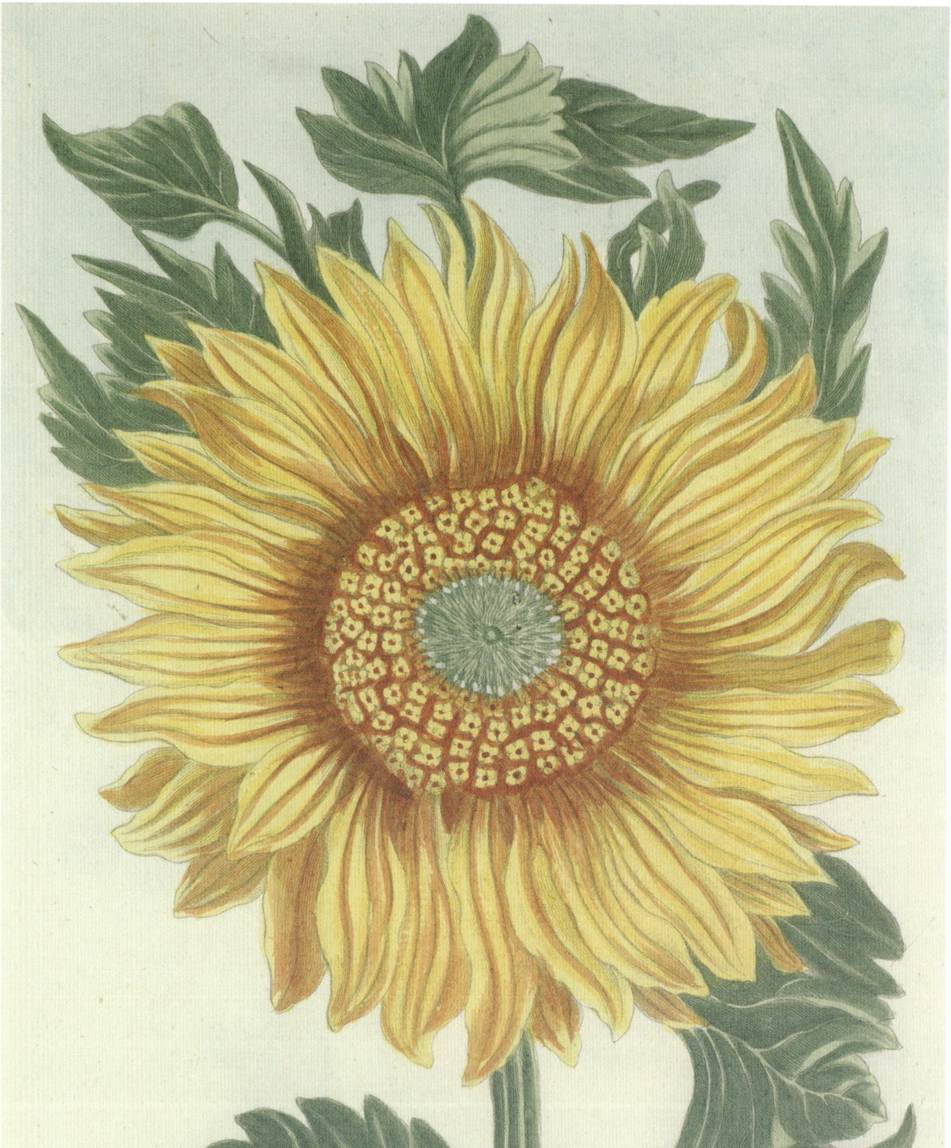

Sunflower (*Helianthus annuus*) by Pierre Joseph Buchoz,
from *Collection Précieuse et Enluminée Des Fleurs...*, Vol. 2, 1776.

Some plants have the power to clean things up

Contaminated soil, getting to grips with

It's not uncommon to find some level of heavy metal contamination in garden soil, especially in cities, which can be caused by historical industry, mining, busy roads and waste disposal. You may not need to fix this if you're only growing flowers (though some plants will not be happy). If you want to grow fruit or veg, though, raised beds avoid the entire issue, while not tackling the actual problem. One solution that does is to grow plants known as hyperaccumulators.

These plants have the superpower of being able to remove heavy metals from contaminated soils via a process called phytoextraction, where metals are absorbed by the roots and then concentrated in the leaves and shoots. The plants are then harvested and removed, thus 'cleaning' the soil, or at least reducing the contamination. It's a technique that can be used on both large and small scales. Hundreds of thousands of sunflowers were planted after the Chernobyl nuclear blast because they have the capacity to absorb radioactive isotopes such as Cesium-137 and Strontium-90. Indeed, sunflowers are often used on new community garden sites as they also can absorb arsenic, chromium, zinc, copper and manganese.

Plants can specialize in just one or more metals, though some, such as willows and many ferns and grasses, can absorb a wide range. It's not all about toxins, either. There is an unusual practice called phytomining, which is when plants are used to extract the likes of, say, gold from a site. The plant is then harvested and the metal extracted. Eucalyptus, for instance, can draw gold from deep in the ground and, in this way, act as a sort of messenger indicating gold deposits.

Here's what to plant to counter those vehicle emissions

Road pollution, alleviating

The secret weapon of a hedge, in terms of sucking up pollution and noise, is its leaves. Studies show that hedges can cut exposure to traffic pollutants by more than 50 per cent. They beat fences for this because leaf surfaces, when added together, make for a much larger area altogether. This, plus the fact that hedges will be deeper than fences, means they are much more effective at trapping pollutants and particularly the tiny, dust-like particles from vehicle exhausts. They can also absorb noise, though studies differ on how much, with a general figure of 6–9 decibels.

All leaves trap some form of air pollutants, but the ones that trap the most are those that are hairy, waxy, scaly or rough. If you live on a busy road, and want to plant a hedge to mop up air pollutants, it makes sense to pay attention to which leaves will give you the best results. Hairy leaves (such as those of *Cotoneaster franchetii*) can capture particles on both sides, with the particles getting trapped between the hairs. Waxy leaves (such as yew or holly) trap and embed the particles. Scaly, overlapping leaves (such as those of red cedar) provide a rough surface that traps a higher number of particles. Rough leaves, such as hawthorn, trap particles on their ridges and surface furrows.

The best hedge of all, a super-hedge if you will, is *Cotoneaster franchetii*. An RHS study found that a 1-m (3-ft) length of *C. franchetii* hedge could, in seven days, trap the same amount of pollution that a car emits over 800km (500 miles). The species trapped 20 per cent more than other species due to its complex leaves. It is also evergreen and so works hard all year round. Any hedge, though, is better than none and the one that is going to fight air pollution and noise the most will be dense and about 1m (3ft) deep by 2m (6ft) high. Your air will be cleaner and quieter. Result.

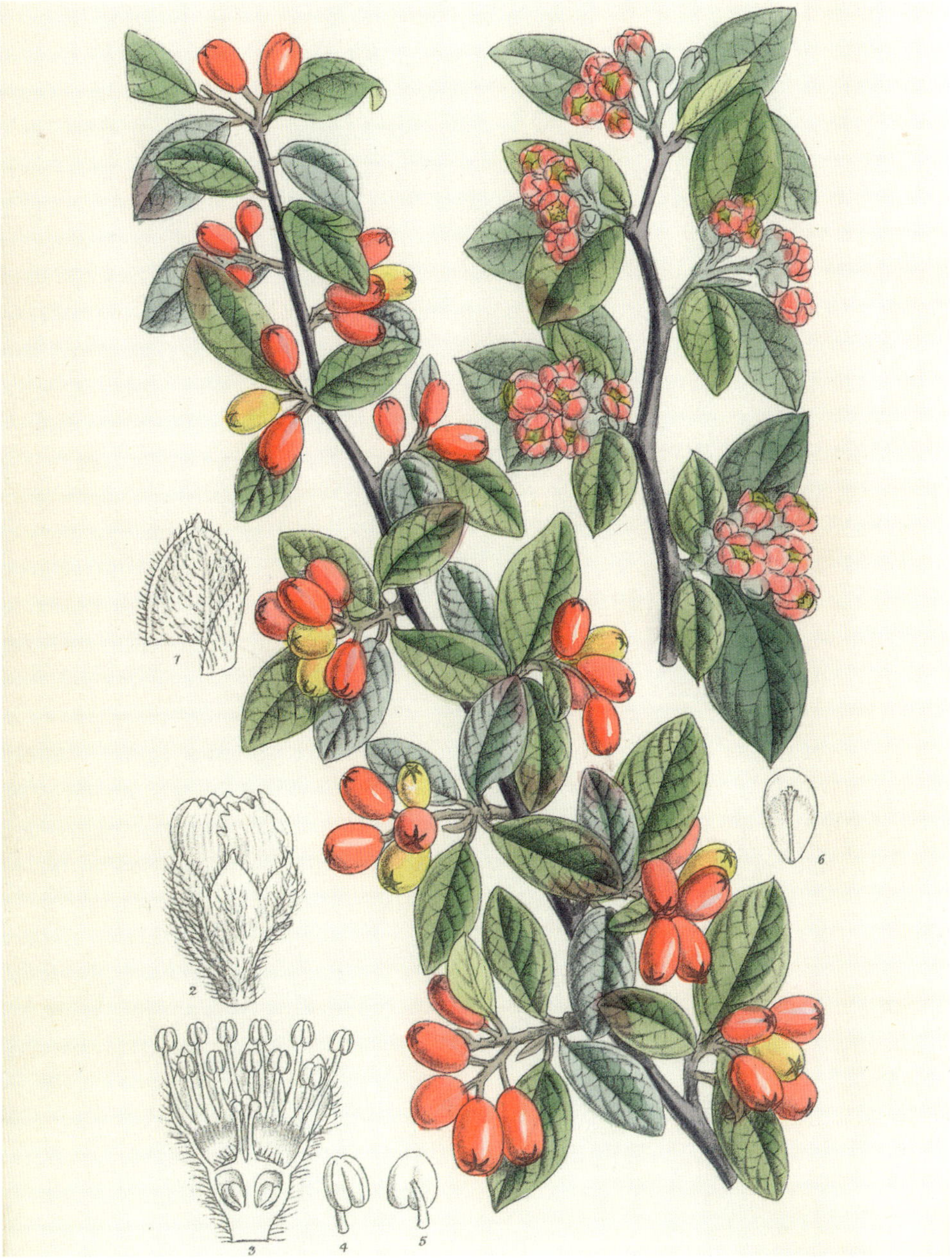

Cotoneaster franchetii, published in *Curtis's Botanical Magazine*, 1914.

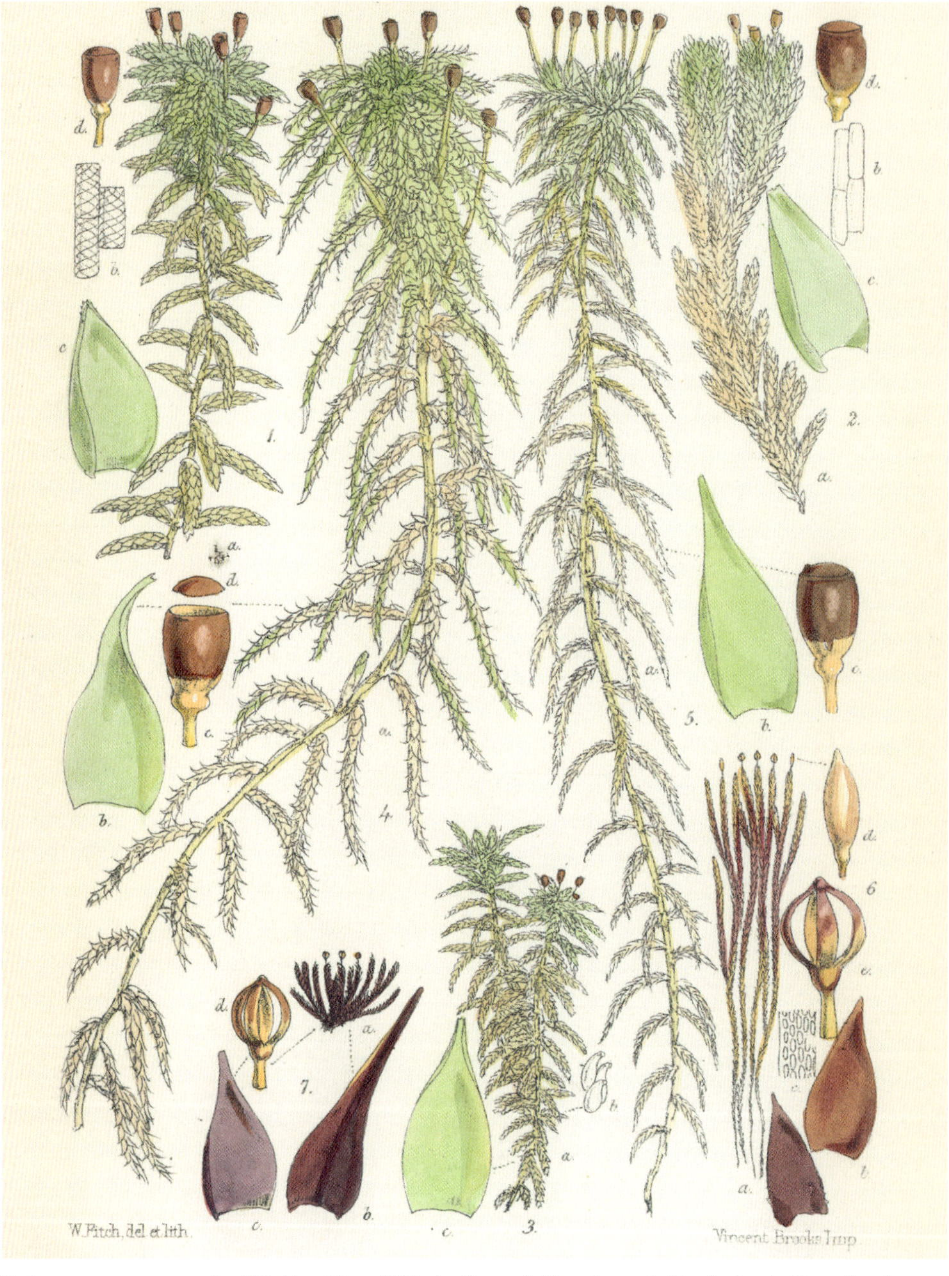

Sphagnum mosses by Walter Hood Fitch, from Miles Joseph Berkeley's *Handbook of British Mosses: Comprising All That Are Known to be Natives of the British Isles*, 1863.

Here's one thing that you must NOT do to make a difference

Save the planet, desire to

Sometimes the subject of peatlands can seem complicated but perhaps less so if you call them bogs, fens and swamps. These are very wet areas in open land; that is, without trees. Nature is on a go-slow here: because it is so wet and acidic, the dead plant matter (mostly sphagnum moss) takes a very long time to decompose. Just 1mm of peat is formed over the course of a year. That means 1m (3ft) of peat takes an incredible 1,000 years to be created. The sheer slowness of this process explains why peatlands store more carbon than all the world's forests. They cover just 3 per cent of the world's surface but account for 30 per cent of all soil carbon.

For those who want to save the planet, the battle to retain carbon, whether it is stored in the ground or tree or plant, is the game-changer. A large-scale cure needs government action as only 17 per cent of peatlands around the world are protected. There is also no clear timescale for banning the sale of peat for horticultural use. Our purchases of peat compost, in the year of 2020 alone, according to the UK's Woodland Trust, could have released 880,000 tonnes of carbon dioxide. That's the equivalent in emissions to driving to the moon and back 4,600 times.

The garden cure is clear cut. You can save the planet, one compost bag at a time. Just don't buy it. It's sounds almost too simple. If you don't buy, peat will stay in bogs, not bags. Instead, buy a bag of peat-free compost – luckily nowadays there's plenty of choice.

'The garden cure is clear cut. You can save the planet, one compost bag at a time.'

Plant a tree, though not all trees are created equal

Save the planet, in a big way

It's photosynthesis that provides the magic when it comes to carbon and trees. During this process, they take in carbon dioxide, water and sunlight and produce oxygen and glucose. The latter provides the tree with the energy it needs to grow, while the carbon remains stored in its trunk, branches and roots. It's called carbon sequestration and it's vital to our planet.

One garden cure for saving the planet is to plant a tree. If you do, that tree will store carbon and, on average, that is estimated to be 10kg (22lb) per year for the first 20 years. If you have some room, then plant a large tree or two. Factors that increase carbon storage include trees that grow fast, live for a long time, and have larger trunks and denser wood. Think Douglas fir (*Pseudotsuga menziesii*), oak (*Quercus*), horse chestnut (*Aesculus hippocastanum*), blue spruce (*Picea pungens*), tulip tree (*Liriodendron tulipifera*), London plane (*Platanus* × *hispanica*) and even dogwood (*Cornus*). The superstar when it comes to carbon is the mangrove (12.3kg/27lb a year), but your average mangrove, which only grows in sub-tropical and tropical climates, often in the water, may not fit into your garden.

'One garden cure for saving the planet is to plant a tree.'

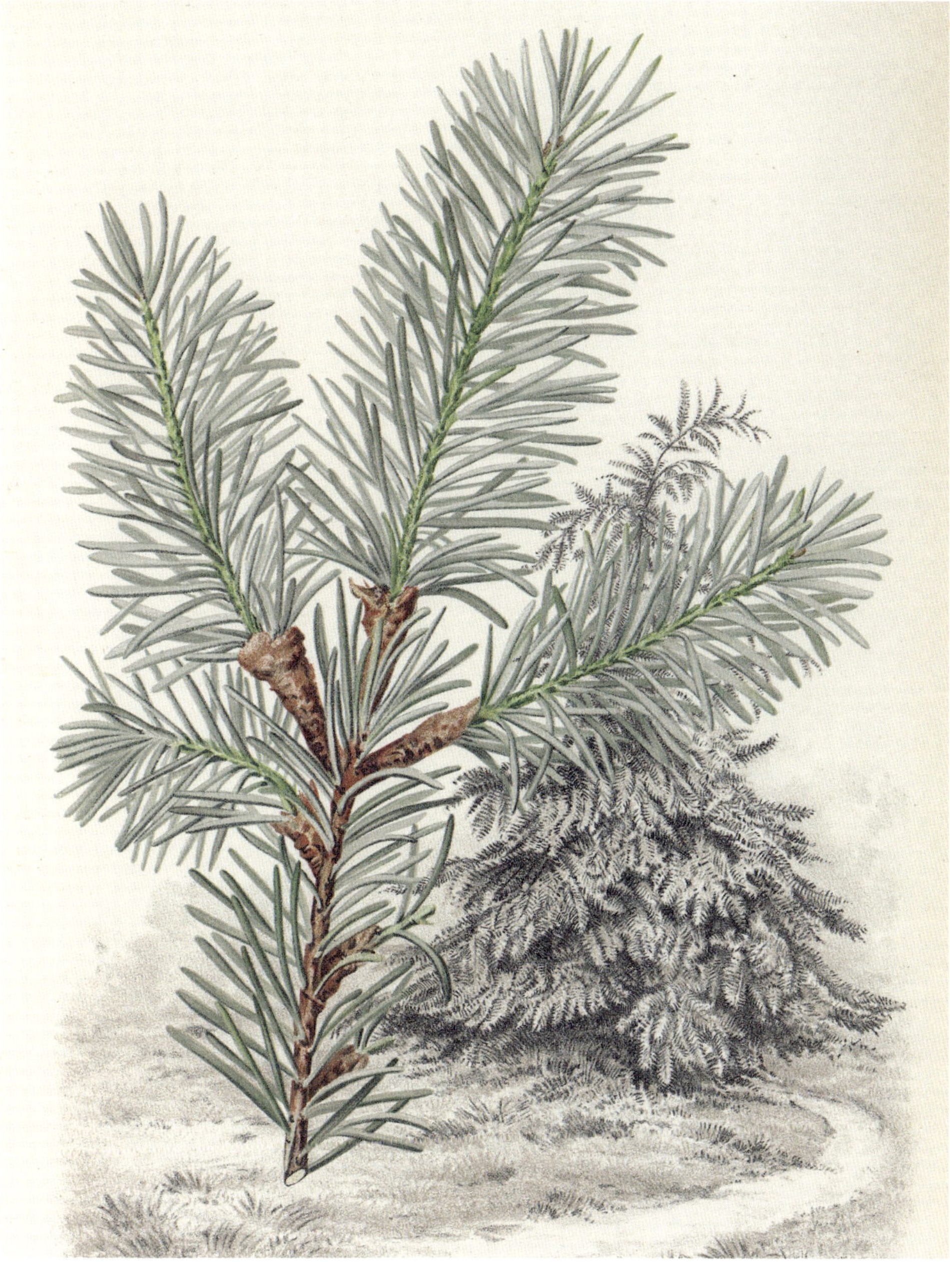

Douglas fir (*Pseudotsuga menziesii*), from the publication *Revue Horticole*, Vol. 67, 1895.

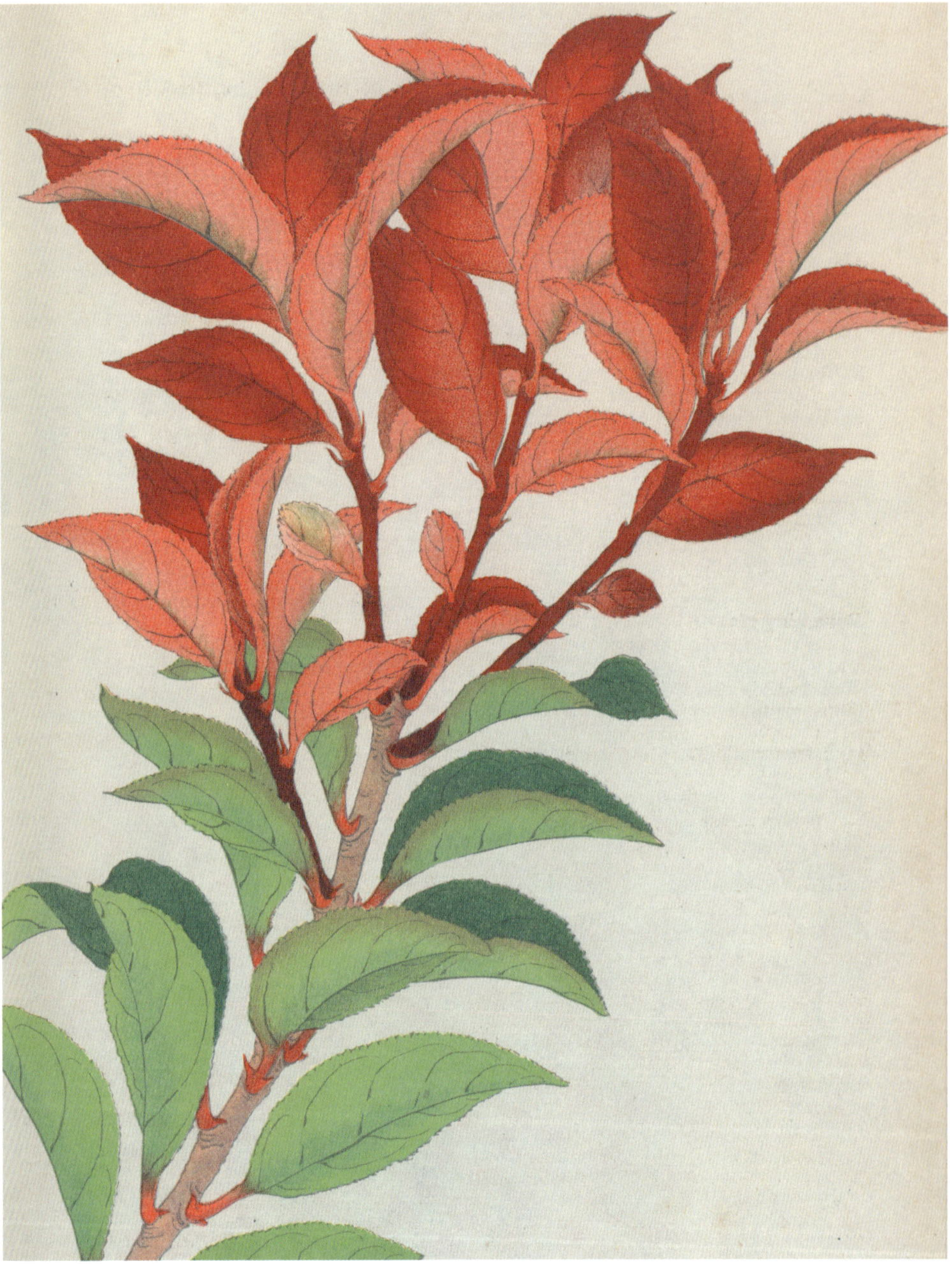

Photinia glabra 'Rubens', from the 'Yokohama Nursery Company Catalogue', 1904.

If you don't have room for a tree, then read on

Save the planet, in small(er) ways

If you remain anxious about saving the planet, or possibly even more so because you don't have room for a tree (see previous cure), then rest assured that it's not only trees that store carbon. If you don't have the room, or the inclination, for a tree, then opt for another plant. As a rule, anything with a woody stem will store more carbon than one with a green stem. Think shrub and, if possible, a longer lasting one, such as *Photinia*. The next step down would be perennials, as they last longer than annuals. Another option is to think of greener substitutions when it comes to other garden projects. If you are thinking of a fence, why not plant a hedge instead? Hedges are beautiful, store carbon and attract wildlife. Win, win, win.

It's time to get drastic with plastic

Save the planet, making a pledge to

Plastic is cheap, durable and lightweight. It's also ubiquitous, with more than 400–460 million tonnes produced every year globally. Most of that is single use and less than 10 per cent is being recycled. Its production is equally problematic as it is mainly from fossil fuels and has doubled in two decades. It's projected to triple by 2060. It's hard not to conclude that we are addicted to plastic and, if we want to save the planet, that's a problem for everyone.

The cure sounds simple: no new plastic. Take a rough inventory of your current plastic, both in the house and garden. Then figure out how to stop there. Reuse, recycle, repurpose but don't buy new. That is easier said than done. In the garden, that means tackling the issue of plastic pots (which take 400 years to break down) with your garden centre and also asking if they'll recycle compost bags. Use wooden seed trays, empty toilet paper rolls and newspaper seed pots. Expect a little bit of failure and celebrate any success. Do this on repeat – inside and outside, as a daily challenge. You'll feel better.

Learn some lessons of life from gastropods

Role model, need for one

You may think you don't like slugs and that may be true, as most people (and especially gardeners) have fraught, if not murderous, feelings towards them. If we see things in a clear-eyed way, though, slugs are much more than a pest that drives you mad by eating your hostas. They are, in so many other ways, the ultimate survivors. Here are some things to admire about slugs...

Flexibility. All terrestrial slugs evolved from terrestrial snails (who were themselves originally marine). This seems to have been about 350 million to 250 million years ago during the Age of Amphibians. Slugs gained something vital by ditching the shells – mobility. Snails have that cumbersome house on their backs and, by their nature, must spend a lot of time 'at home'. Slugs can move with the groove, squeezing through all sorts of cracks and crannies (they can stretch to 20 times thinner), as well as underground into pores and earthworm burrows.

Slugs protect themselves. The big issue (other than all humans trying to kill them) is the sun. Slugs don't want to dry out, which is why they spend most of the day underground or under leaves. Their secret weapon is their slime, which puts off many predators and, if they encounter danger, such as a slug pellet, they can even produce more mucous to try and slime it off, so to speak. They can use their tentacles to smell slime trails, recognize their own (which means they can go back to their favourite leaf pile, or wherever), and tell if other slime trails were made by their own species.

Slugs like each other – and show it. All slugs are hermaphrodites, which means they have both male and female organs. Many can self-fertilize. They don't need each other to have their endless slugettes or, to use the correct term, neonates. But slugs aren't selfish. They want to connect. Slug courtship is not, as you'd expect, a quick affair. Take the grey field slug: first the slugs need to find a partner, often by following a slime trail. The pair will circle each other for up to an hour, stroking each other with a special appendage. This is the slug equivalent of foreplay. Both then turn out their genitalia and lock them together. Drops of sperm are traded. It will be a few days before they (yes, each of them) will lay their eggs, in a

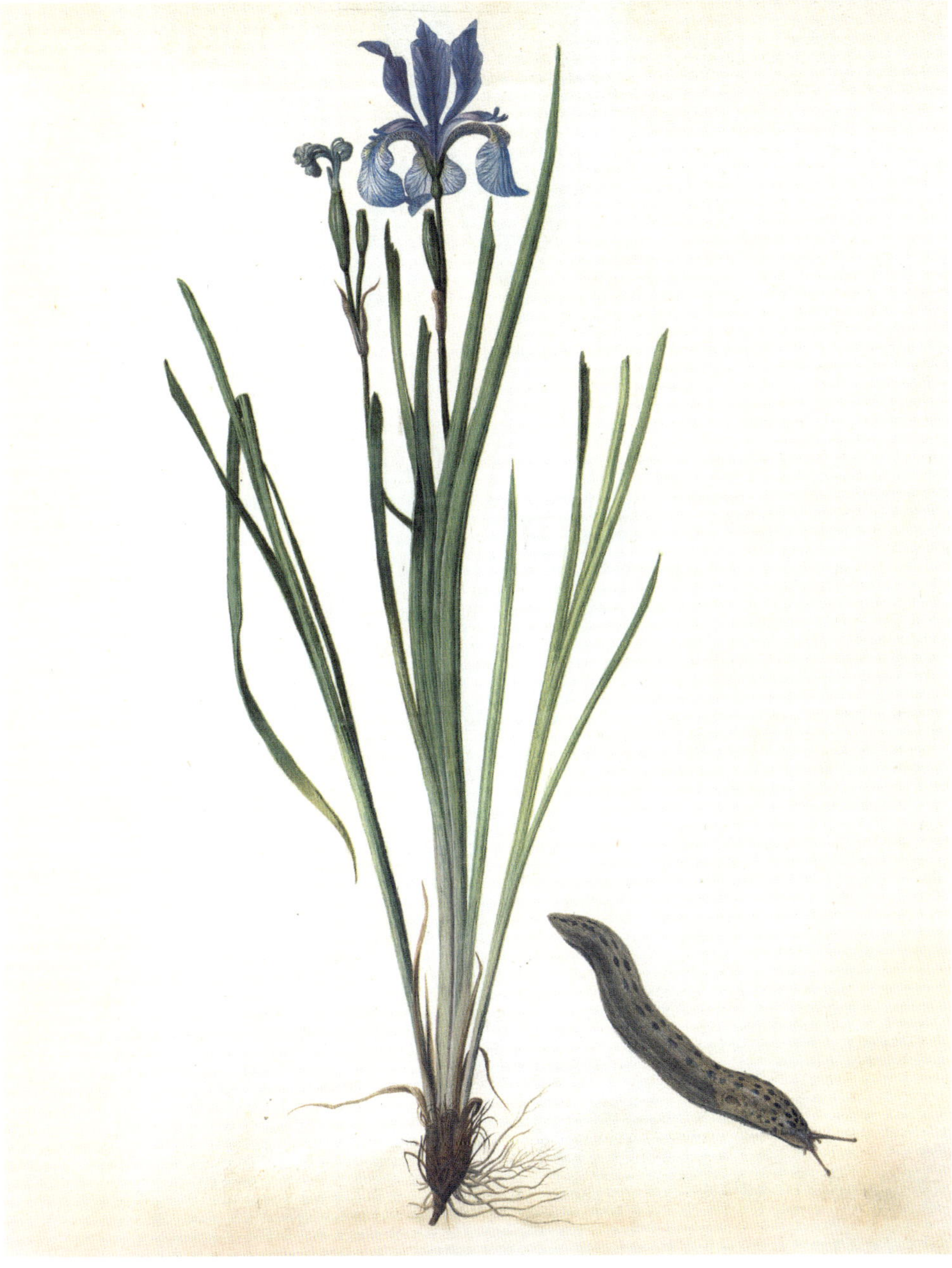

Siberian flag (*Iris sibirica*) and slug, watercolour on paper by
Pieter van Kouwenhoorn from his album of paintings, 1630s.

small hole which will hatch in one or two weeks. Slugs that live for just six months can produce some seven hundred eggs. (No wonder there are so many in your garden.)

Slugs are diligent eaters. Anyone with a hosta knows that slugs have an appetite, but they do not live to eat. They need to eat a lot (all that slow moving burns up calories), and that means up to twice their body weight a day. What, exactly, they eat depends on their species. Options include plants, detritus, earthworms and, for some, all of those. They won't overeat, though. They eat to live, not the other way around.

Slugs might think (if they could) that they are paranoid, but in general we really all are out to get them. Most of us do not think slugs are 'cute', as we do snails. We may even be able to eat snails if they are called escargot, but slugs are very rarely, if ever, on the menu. We have devised an array of weapons, including beer traps and rings of eggshells or grit, to wound them. Other strategies involve copper tape, wool, garlic and chilli. It's not clear what really works, though you can remove them, physically, by taking them at least 20m (65ft) away.

Our obsession with getting rid of slugs doesn't negate the fact that, actually, we can learn a lot from them. They are the ultimate survivors, slow but steady, flexible, caring and also fantastic garden recyclers. In their own way, they really could be role models.

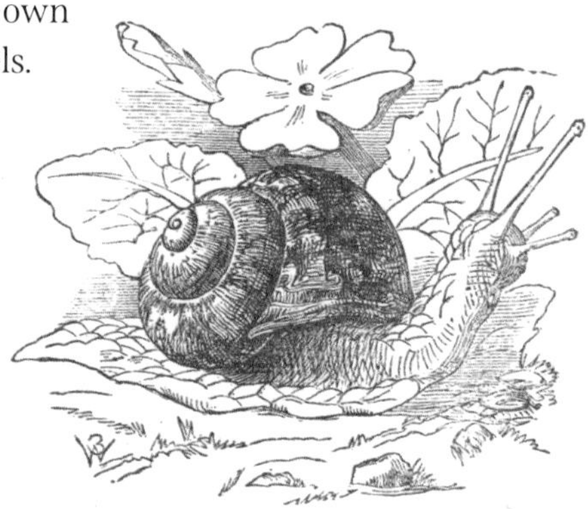

Snail by Sara Wood, from *The Dwellers in Our Gardens: Their Lives and Works*, 1877.

The Lindley Library Treasures

The illustrations in this book come from the RHS Lindley Library's superb botanical collection of some 30,000 artworks and over 2,500 rare books. The collections span more than 500 years of horticultural history and include many rare drawings, paintings and printed works, the most valued of which are referred to here as 'The Treasures'. They include works by Elizabeth Blackwell, Claude Aubriet and Caroline Maria Applebee. All feature in this book, along with those by many other noteworthy artists.

The library holds a complete set of *A Curious Herbal* by **Elizabeth Blackwell** (1699–1758). The volumes include 500 of her meticulous illustrations, which were first published between 1737 and 1739 in weekly instalments. Blackwell drew from living plants at London's Chelsea Physic Garden, enabling her readers (which included doctors and apothecaries) to gain an understanding of their medical uses and effects. (For more about her personal story, see pages 191–2.)

French artist **Claude Aubriet** (*c*.1665–1742) was a botanical illustrator at the Jardin du Roi in Paris who, in 1707, was appointed as royal botanical painter. He brought a new level of scientific rigour to depicting members of the plant kingdom. The library holds 668 pen and ink drawings by Aubriet, plus eight watercolours and gouache on vellum.

The work of English artist **Caroline Maria Applebee** (*c*.1787–1854) provides a vivid record of the flowers that were fashionable during the Victorian period. The collection includes 324 watercolour paintings of flowers such as rhododendrons and camellias which were then novelties to British gardeners. Her later work, unheralded in its day, concentrated on the Victoriana obsessions of fuchsias and pelargoniums.

The RHS Lindley Library is located at 80 Vincent Square in London SW1P 2PE. Scan this QR code to explore more than 500 years of gardening history and science on RHS Digital Collections.

Acknowledgements This book has been a labour of love and has only been possible because of the encouragement of Alison Starling, Publishing Director of Octopus Books (which includes Mitchell Beazley), and the outstanding team at the Royal Horticultural Society. I am especially grateful to Helen Griffin, RHS Books Publisher, who came to me with the idea and has been enthusiastically supportive throughout the process. The amazing RHS Lindley Library in Vincent Square in London holds a wealth of artistic botanical treasures but, of course, they all needed to be found and digitized: deep thanks go to Crestina Forcina, Digital Collections Assistant, and Mark Hobbs, Digital Collections Manager. Thanks to RHS Books Editor Simon Maughan for his key advice, Mike Grant, RHS Contributing Editor, Specialist Publications, for his botanical expertise, and to Chief Entomologist Hayley Jones, for her guidance. At Mitchell Beazley I am grateful for the skilled editing of Leanne Bryan, Senior Editor, as well as the care and attention to detail of Copyeditor Caroline West. Art Director Juliette Norsworthy has made this endeavour into a thing of beauty. Friends have helped me out during this process in all sorts of ways and, in particular, I would like to acknowledge Sandra Parsons, Vicky Wilson and Tom Neville. Finally, I owe a great deal to my own garden, which teaches me something new almost every day.

The Royal Horticultural Society is the UK's leading gardening charity dedicated to advancing horticulture and promoting good gardening. Its charitable work includes providing expert advice and information in print, online and at its five major gardens and annual shows, training gardeners of every age, creating hands-on opportunities for children to grow plants, and sharing research into plants, wildlife, wellbeing and environmental issues affecting gardeners. For more information, visit: www.rhs.org.uk or call 020 3176 5800.

Ann Treneman writes the Notebook column for Saturday's *The Times* and is the newspaper's gardening columnist. She was previously its chief theatre critic and award-winning parliamentary sketch writer and feature writer. Ann grew up in Oregon in the US, but is now British and American. She splits her time between London and the seaside in Kent, and views 'having fun' as one of life's essentials. She is the author of *RHS Greener Guides: Containers* and *RHS Horti Curious* (both published by Mitchell Beazley). She designed a show garden for RHS Chelsea Flower Show in 2022.

Index

First published in Great Britain in 2026
by Mitchell Beazley, an imprint of
Octopus Publishing Group Ltd, in association
with the Royal Horticultural Society
Carmelite House
50 Victoria Embankment
London EC4Y 0DZ
www.octopusbooks.co.uk

An Hachette UK Company
www.hachette.co.uk

The authorized representative in the EEA is
Hachette Ireland, 8 Castlecourt Centre, Dublin 15,
D15 XTP3, Ireland (email: info@hbgi.ie)

Copyright © Royal Horticultural Society Enterprises
Limited 2026

Distributed in the US by Hachette Book Group
1290 Avenue of the Americas, 4th and 5th Floors
New York, NY 10104

Distributed in Canada by Canadian Manda Group
664 Annette St., Toronto, Ontario, Canada M6S 2C8

All rights reserved. No part of this work may be
reproduced or utilized in any form or by any means,
electronic or mechanical, including photocopying,
recording or by any information storage and
retrieval system, without the prior written
permission of the publisher.

The rights of Ann Treneman to be identified as the
Author of this work have been asserted under
the Copyright, Designs and Patents Act 1988.

ISBN: 978-1-84601-680-6
eISBN: 978-1-84601-681-3

A CIP catalogue record for this book is available
from the British Library.

Printed and bound in China.

10 9 8 7 6 5 4 3 2 1

For Mitchell Beazley
Publishing Director: Alison Starling
Senior Editor: Leanne Bryan
Art Director: Juliette Norsworthy
Designer: Ella McLean
Copyeditor: Caroline West
Assistant Production Manager: Lisa Pinnell

For the RHS
RHS Books Publisher: Helen Griffin
RHS Consultant Editors: Simon Maughan
and Mike Grant
RHS Head of Editorial: Tom Howard
RHS Lindley Library: Mark Hobbs and
Crestina Forcina

MIX
Paper | Supporting responsible forestry
FSC
www.fsc.org
FSC® C008047

Additional picture credits
Pages 1, 43: © Lilian Snelling/RHS/Originally
commissioned by Henry John Elwes; Pages 7, 100, 131,
184: © Valerie Finnis/RHS Lindley Collections; Page
17: © Evelyn Dunbar Estate; Page 123: © Raffaello
Bencini. All rights reserved 2026/Bridgeman Images

Disclaimer

This book is a reference book about the history of plants and their uses. The information in this book is for informational purposes and any recipes or treatments within it are for reference purposes only. This book is not intended as a replacement for professional medical treatment and should not be relied upon as recommending, encouraging or promoting any specific diet or practice. It is also not intended as a guide to which plants are edible or have nutritional or medicinal benefits or to replace the advice of a nutritionist, physician or qualified medical practitioner.

We strongly advise you to consult a medical practitioner before using any herbal remedies, especially if you have an existing medical condition, are taking medication, are pregnant or are breast-feeding. You should not use the information in this book as a substitute for diagnosis, medication or other treatments prescribed by a qualified medical practitioner.

There is the possibility of allergic or other adverse reactions from the use of any plants mentioned (and plants not mentioned) in this book. You should seek the advice of your doctor or other qualified health provider with any questions you may have, especially in relation to medical conditions or allergies. Some plants may interact with prescription drugs, including, but not limited to, the Pill and antidepressants; if you are using any medication, you should always consult with a qualified medical practitioner before taking any herbal remedies.

The publishers and author do not accept any liability for any harm that results from your use, or misuse, of this book, or for your failure to seek appropriate medical advice.

Royalties from the sale of this book are received by RHS Enterprises Limited which pays over all of its profits to the RHS, as parent charity, and so inspires passion and excellence in horticulture.